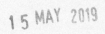

THE NEWBORN IDENTITY

Revelations from the first year of parenting

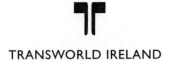

twisteddoodles

TRANSWORLD IRELAND

www.penguin.co.uk

FOR ALL THE PARENTS WHO AREN'T SURE WHAT THEY ARE DOING BUT ARE DOING THE BEST THEY CAN.

TRANSWORLD IRELAND
Penguin Random House Ireland,
Morrison Chambers, 32 Nassau Street, Dublin 2, Ireland
www.transworldireland.ie

Transworld Ireland is part of the Penguin Random House group of companies whose addresses can be found at global.penguinrandomhouse.com

Penguin
Random House
UK

First published in the UK and Ireland in 2019
by Transworld Ireland
an imprint of Transworld Publishers

Copyright © Maria Boyle 2019

Maria Boyle has asserted her right under the Copyright, Designs and Patents Act 1988 to be identified as the author of this work.

A CIP catalogue record for this book
is available from the British Library.

ISBN 9781848272583

Typeset in 10/13pt Gotham Book by Julia Lloyd Design
Printed and bound in Great Britain by Clays Ltd, Elcograf S.p.A.

Penguin Random House is committed to a sustainable future for our business, our readers and our planet. This book is made from Forest Stewardship Council® certified paper.

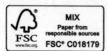

MIX
Paper from
responsible sources
FSC® C018179

1 3 5 7 9 10 8 6 4 2

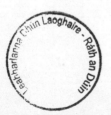

CONTENTS

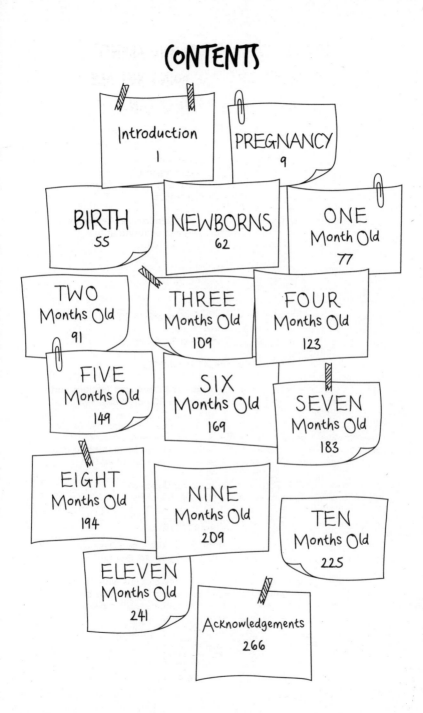

INTRODUCTION

When I was young I didn't want to be a mother, I wanted to be a zoo keeper – or maybe a vet. Once, an episode of *Blue Peter* asked children to draw what they imagined they would be doing when they were thirty years old. I'd always loved drawing so I drew myself as a vet – a single vet who owned a German Shepherd and a parrot. There was no husband, there were no children.

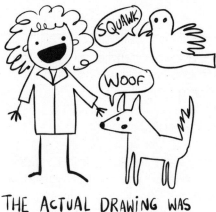

THE ACTUAL DRAWING WAS
BETTER THAN THIS

I am eighteen years old and in university when I have my first kiss. He is a friend I've come to know better through writing emails to each other; the things we couldn't say, we wrote. He found me attractive and that was crazy to me – that getting to know me through writing and me being funny was attractive.

I am single and in Dublin doing my PhD in science. I know no one and it is lonely because this isn't my city and I am tired of spending my evenings reading in the

1

tiny room I'm renting. I use a dating site to make friends and meet a man and he is from Dublin. He has a beard and glasses and I find him funny and attractive and he doesn't kiss me.

However, he asks to meet me for coffee after work the next day and we feed pigeons and talk in a café. He walks me to my bus and as it arrives he asks to kiss me and he does. It is the best first kiss I ever have.

Nine years later we are talking with two of his friends and one of them asks, 'When are you getting married?'

'Next year,' my boyfriend replies.

'Next year?' I repeat.

'Yes.'

'OK, shake on it.'

And he shakes my hand and I go to the bathroom. On the toilet, I realize something and rush back.

'I meant that!' I say.

'So did I.'

'We're engaged?'

'We are.'

I burst into tears and kiss him. His friends look confused, not realizing that within a week we'll have the venue booked.

We got married in Dublin Zoo because I may not have become a zoo keeper but I found a keeper there.

Once we got married, people started wondering about babies. They kept staring at my tummy. Either that or they were checking to see whether I'd put the weight back on that I'd lost for my wedding. If I went out and didn't drink they'd think that I was pregnant, and if I did drink they'd think that I was pregnant and a terrible parent.

The thing is, lots of my friends already had babies. I couldn't remember their babies' names, which wasn't so bad as the babies couldn't remember them either.

2

WARNING: THIS DRAWING CONTAINS SCENES OF AN ADULT NATURE!

we're married

I WANT TO START A PENSION

I GOT US A RESCUE CAT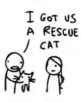

WHAT ARE YOU READING? THE NEWS

THESE ARE ALL BILLS! WHO IS HE!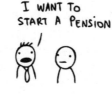

I'm PREGNANT! I DID THAT

YOU OWN A HOUSE! NEGATIVE EQUITY HERE WE COME

WHAT COULD POSSIBLY GO WRONG! VOTING

WHY ARE WE HAVING CAKE FOR BREAKFAST? BECAUSE WE'RE ADULTS AND WE CAN!

However, I also couldn't remember whether they'd had a boy or a girl, so I'd ask, 'How's the wee one?' And you knew it was probably fine, doing things I couldn't relate to – except for crying for no apparent reason. Sometimes my friends might ask me to hold their baby, which I didn't want to, in case it exploded in my hands or cried. In which case, the only instruction was to 'support the head', as if it were a football team.

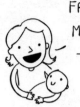

THIS BABY IS SO SMALL AND
FRAGILE BUT THEY'RE THE
MOST IMPORTANT THING IN
THE WORLD, MY EVERYTHING...

WOULD YOU LIKE
TO HOLD HIM?

Huh? Sorry....
I just dropped
my phone...

A person's interest in pregnancy and babies seems to follow a trend, which goes from interested to uninterested to interested, according to the age of the mother.

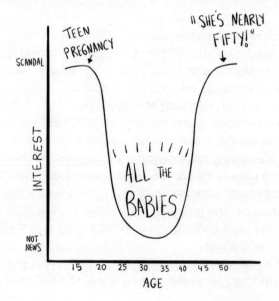

After we married I wanted to avoid having babies, so life could be our adventure a little bit longer, before we finally said, 'Yes, we are having babies.' I believed we weren't ready to become parents – I was barely able to parent myself – but time moves on.

WHAT I THOUGHT WOULD HAPPEN BEFORE WE HAD KIDS

- ☐ Learn to drive
- ☐ Get promotion
- ☐ Buy a house

WHAT ACTUALLY HAPPENED?

- ☑ None of the above: we just got older.

To be honest, I had pretty much convinced myself I couldn't have children. An idea compounded by my periods showing up whenever they thought I'd like a social occasion ruined, and time spent poring over the side effects of drugs I'd been given back when I had cancer as a teenager, had me thinking that.

When I was an overweight fifteen-year-old, I had three things – huge glasses, a ginger mushroom-bob haircut and cancer – and chemo got rid of only one of them. Mercifully, not losing my hair meant I didn't have to tell people I'd cancer, because my appearance attracted enough unwanted attention as it was. I didn't want to also be 'the girl who has cancer' or 'the girl who has a 20 per cent chance of surviving'. I just wanted to figure out who I was.

After a few years that percentage increased. I wasn't 'the girl who had survived cancer', I was the girl who had a PhD, who worked as a scientist, who was an artist and a wife, but I didn't know if I could be a mother.

I also didn't know whether I *should* have children. My malignant melanoma had progressed rapidly until it got to stage 3, and after the surgery and treatments the only thing the doctors seemed to give it was time. Time spent waiting to see if it would come back.

They didn't say to me, 'Congratulations, you don't have cancer any more. You're free to live your life as you please.' It was more, 'It's been five years since you had it.' And then it was ten.

I remember my oncologist telling me not to have any children until I'd been in remission for ten years. At the time, children weren't even on my horizon. However, at my final appointment, I asked him if he'd said that because treatment during pregnancy might put the baby at risk. He replied that it was because he didn't want a child to be left without its mother. I realize how heavy that sounds but he didn't mean to be cruel, and at the time it didn't feel that way either. It was just a fact.

I live under the shadow of having had cancer. It's not something that I actively think about, but it has affected how I live my life. When you're a teenager, I think you're meant to feel a bit invincible. I'd peeked behind the curtain, though. I knew I was mortal.

Even now, no one can tell me for certain that the cancer won't come back. Even though I've put many years and many experiences between that time and now, I've found it difficult to commit to long-term goals because I don't know what might happen in a year's – or five years' – time. It felt incredibly daunting to bring a husband into that uncertainty – never mind children – because in the back of my mind there was a voice that was saying, 'Maybe the cancer is waiting to come back when I've got much more to lose.'

Starting to commit to things – even something as simple as getting a cat – felt scary and made me anxious but then I got married because I was trying to push myself forward into the uncertainty. If I didn't, the cancer might not have taken my life, but it would have taken my capacity to live it.

So now I'm married and we're having a conversation about having children and I'm saying I want to give it a go. Then, you find yourself having sex, with the idea of maybe wanting kids. You're trying for a kid, but you're still having sex, you're still killing time because the cinema isn't for two hours and it's a good idea. But you aren't telling anyone that this is happening.

WHAT THEY SAY....

We are trying for a baby!

WHAT I HEAR...

We are having a lot of unprotected sex.

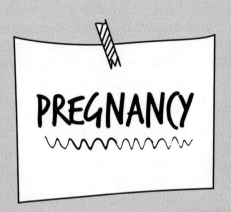

15 October 2014

My period is late, a fact I informed my husband Colm of at 2 a.m. I suggested that maybe we should go to a 24-hour supermarket to buy a pregnancy test. Sensibly, he said 'no' and I lay in bed, worried that I was pregnant, because although I wanted it, it felt too soon and I thought about how much our lives would change.

   I wasn't ready. I took a test. It was negative.

20 October

My period came. My initial relief was followed by sadness; sadness and a realization that I don't think I'll ever feel ready but maybe I'll never get the chance to.

16 November

Yesterday, Colm and I flew to London for his brother's wedding and today I have to catch a flight to France for a conference. I think this should make me feel like an international jet-setter but mostly I feel tired.

20 November

I'm back from the conference. It was nice to meet people and talk about science. I met a doctor there who told me about her daughters and showed me photos. She asked if I wanted kids. I told her I did but that I don't think it will happen.

23 November

I went out with a friend of mine, got drunk and complained that I couldn't get pregnant because I keep having conversations about it.

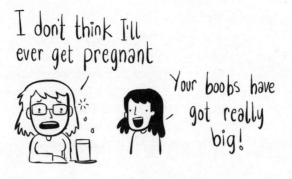

'It's because I'm due my period,' I say, telling her not to be looking at my boobs.

27 November

I found out I am pregnant because I peed on a stick on Monday. I also peed on my hand, but mostly on the stick. It was a test left over from last month's pregnancy freak-out. For some reason I thought that pregnancy tests would be all certainty and shout 'YOU'RE PREGNANT' at you, if that were the case. It was negative. I put it in the bin in the bathroom.

Yesterday morning I fished it out. There was a faint line. I went out for more tests and took another two – both were positive. I was all the emotions, I wanted to hug someone. I stared at the cat. I didn't hug her.

Colm is working in a job he hates. He came home late, looking defeated.

'How are you?' I asked.

'Tired. How are you?'

'Pregnant.'

He was shocked; he is delighted.

WHEN I FOUND OUT I WAS PREGNANT
I USED A CHEAP TEST!

two for a fiver!

I USED BOTH!!
THEN I BOUGHT THE MORE EXPENSIVE
DIGITAL ONES two for
twenty quid!

I didn't n_eed to buy them
but they felt like a scratch card I'd definitely
win on, plus it felt like peeing on a
CASIO WATCH. please
don't —

FIRST TRIMESTER

2 December

We have nicknamed the bump-to-be 'Colm Junior', or CoJu. Mostly so I can speak in code about what's going on, as I'm in pain. CoJu seems to be doing a lot of construction work on my insides. If my womb is rented accommodation I definitely don't think the baby will be getting its deposit back.

6 December

Last night, I did a stand-up comedy gig. Afterwards, I had a bleed and some pain but Colm was away. So I talked to a nurse on the phone who sent me to the maternity hospital, where I sat in the emergency room on my own from midnight to 3 a.m., waiting to be told I was OK and that the baby was OK. I've only been pregnant a week but it suddenly felt as if it were all over.

A scan of my abdomen showed nothing – a possible ectopic pregnancy, the sonographer said. I went for a blood test to check my hormone levels and I've to go back in two days for a follow-up test.

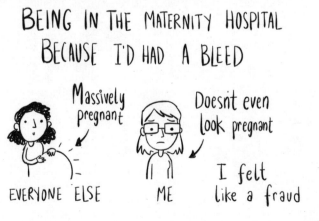

BEING IN THE MATERNITY HOSPITAL BECAUSE I'D HAD A BLEED

Massively pregnant

EVERYONE ELSE

Doesn't even look pregnant

ME

I felt like a fraud

8 December

This morning I went in for the follow-up blood test and at 2 p.m. the hospital called me. I needed to come in for a scan, they said. I couldn't leave work then and there, though – they didn't know. It was another couple of hours before I finally managed to get away. When Colm and I got to the hospital, A&E told us to go to the early pregnancy unit, which was closed by that time. I was finding it hard to hold it together, but eventually A&E saw us, even though we'd gone to them first. As I waited to be scanned, I couldn't stop shaking and my teeth were chattering. Colm was concerned, and asked if I was cold. I wasn't – it was nerves.

The doctor did an internal ultrasound this time.

As she moved the probe around, she said, 'Your hormone levels were pretty high, so I'd expect to see something.'

And I asked, 'Er... could my levels be so high because it's twins?'

'Well, there's one and there's the other.'

I'm only 5 weeks pregnant!

The idea that it might be twins hasn't come from there being a family history or some massive hunch. It's come from my mum saying, 'Either you or your brother is going to have twins.' It sounds a little random, but my mother has been right about other things. For instance:

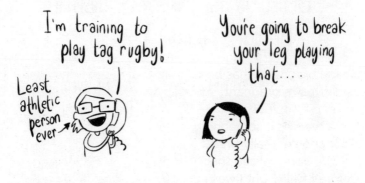

I'm training to play tag rugby!

Least athletic person ever →

You're going to break your leg playing that....

14

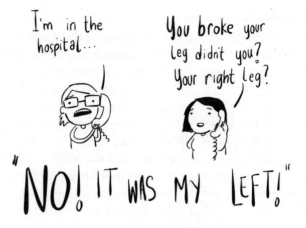

By the time I got pregnant my brother already had a girl and a boy but two years apart, so Colm and I had joked about it.

'Imagine if we were having twins.'

'Oh ho ho, that would be hilarious.'

Well, suddenly it's not a joke. Now I've to hide the fact that I'm pregnant and it's twins.

9 December

CoJu definitely isn't getting their deposit back because the lease on my womb stipulated 'one occupant' and they've moved in a friend we've named 'Maria Junior', or MaJu.

10 December

So far, pregnancy has been a bit of a lonely place. You know you're pregnant, you start to feel it but you have to keep it to yourself.

It feels as if someone has slammed my tits in a car door and I'm really tired.

I've also realized that I spent a number of days before I found out I was pregnant, complaining loudly that my tits hurt. Someone asked then if I could be expecting, and I said no. Today, to throw them off the scent, in the middle of the lab I asked for a sanitary pad at the top of my voice. That'll do it.

13 December

Colm and I are in Sweden to see my brother and his family. He emigrated here in May with his pregnant Swedish girlfriend and my nephew, who is almost three. They had a baby girl and we're here for her baptism – I'm going to be godmother. They live in the middle of nowhere, a town somewhere in the middle of the country, and getting here involved a plane, a train and an automobile.

My brother collects us from the train station and drives us through some of the first snow, joking about how he doesn't have snow tyres yet. At the dinner table, I tell them that I'm pregnant. I'm apprehensive about breaking the news because it's so early, but they're happy for us. I ask them not to tell anyone, especially our parents. My relationship with my mum and dad – with my mum especially – is difficult right now and my brother's isn't much better. Within the space of three years I got married and my brother had a kid and emigrated. I don't know if it's us growing up or what, but relations are fraught these days.

The celebrations are great but the nausea I'm experiencing means that I'm finding it difficult to eat. At the reception there is a massive sandwich cake filled with tuna and mayonnaise, and topped with meats and cheese. It is apparently very tasty but I can't bear to be near it. Someone asks if I'm vegetarian and I say yes, that's the reason I'm avoiding the cake.

I play with my nephew and later make my four-month-old goddaughter laugh so much she poops herself. Before we leave, my sister-in-law gives me a load of maternity clothes she has. The idea that I'll need them at some point feels ridiculous.

16 December

I am 7 weeks pregnant with twins, a fact I have to keep to myself for another five weeks, but it is coming up to Christmas. This is good because it means I will have a week or so off work to deal with the fact that I am incredibly exhausted, developing a compulsion to buy blankets and hoodies to curl up in, and feeling increasingly nauseous. The nausea is bad because Christmas involves a lot of eating, something which I am usually incredibly on board with.

It's believed that pregnancy sickness plays a role in protecting the growing foetus. It's basically like a bouncer stopping you from ingesting anything that could cause harm to you or the baby. This might include meat or fish, which could potentially be carrying bacteria; fruit because...I don't know, I just don't want any fruit. No vegetables, either...No, I'm OK, I don't want any chocolate. Yes, I know it's Christmas...

Suspicion is already on me that I might be pregnant. I'm having to go to some extraordinary lengths to hide it from my work. But our work Christmas party is coming up and in order to avoid it I've had to recruit someone else to embellish my lie. That person is John, someone who is a good friend and who has no problem telling people I have explosive diarrhoea.

24 December

Colm and I were meant to go to my parents' for Christmas this year. We got married last year and spent our first Christmas as a married couple with Colm's parents. One of the reasons for this was because of how much my relationship with my mum has broken down in recent years. We used to be so close – I would tell her everything – and then something changed.

My decision not to get married in a church wouldn't have come as a shock – she said she expected it.

HIDING MY PREGNANCY FROM WORK

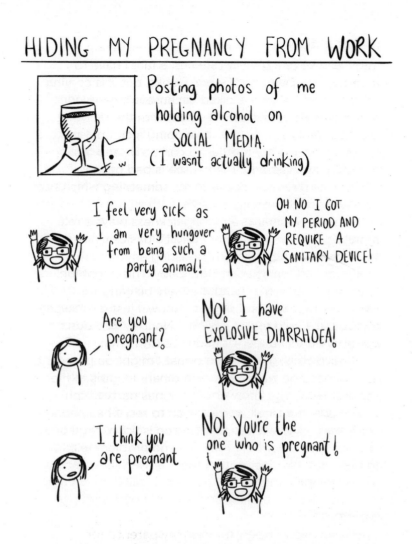

Posting photos of me holding alcohol on SOCIAL MEDIA. (I wasn't actually drinking)

I feel very sick as I am very hungover from being such a party animal!

OH NO I GOT MY PERIOD AND REQUIRE A SANITARY DEVICE!

Are you pregnant?

NO! I have EXPLOSIVE DIARRHOEA!

I think you are pregnant

NO! You're the one who is pregnant!

Initially, she seemed happy for me, but as the day of the wedding drew nearer, the more she pulled away.

The day I got married I didn't get ready with her, and one of the only things she said to me that day was, 'Congratulations, I suppose.'

My dad was caught in the middle. He didn't take sides. He couldn't. He was worried about what was happening to his wife and probably felt unable to

19

resolve it. He looked so happy as he was giving me away, and gave a glowing speech at the reception, praising who Colm and I were. During a moment when I had him on his own, I asked what I could have done differently. He said it wasn't about me, not really.

'You manufacture your own happiness,' he said to me, and told me my mother would find hers again.

After the wedding, I didn't talk to my mother for a while – not directly. I spoke to my dad instead. My dad, in whom I didn't usually confide, with whom I'd had screaming matches as a teenager, who had learned about my life through what I told Mum. Now, he was the conduit to her.

Colm and I married in May, then things between Mum and I came to a head in August. During a phone call every hurt she had poured out, every grievance, and things she would regret saying. I kept my composure but afterwards I cried – it hadn't always been like this.

The thing is, growing up I was really close to my mother. She was the person to whom I told all my problems. She knew about the bullies, the bad boyfriends, the small worries and the big. She's practical and smart – she wanted to be a nurse but worked until she got married, a time at which women were expected to give up their jobs to raise their families. She became a stay-at-home mum and I guess she still is, given that my older sister is autistic and lives at home with my parents.

When I was fifteen, my mum was the one who realized there was something not quite right about a mole on my leg, which eventually turned out to be cancerous.

When we went back to the doctor, after they'd tried unsuccessfully to burn it off, she said, 'It needs to be removed.'

The doctor said, 'I'll refer you to the surgeon and we'll see what he says.'

20

We got to the surgeon and my mother said, 'The GP says this needs to be removed.'

The surgeon said, 'Well, I was going to leave it, but if he's concerned . . .'

This kickstarted a chain of events and I was soon diagnosed with cancer. It was on my leg, which was fine, but then it spread and things got more real.

By lying, she essentially saved my life.

However, when I got older and moved away, I told her about my problems less. Then, when I started to see a counsellor, perhaps she thought that meant that I didn't need her any more. That wasn't the case – I just felt broken in a way she couldn't fix.

People tell me that I am brave when I talk about having had cancer but it is mostly because I shield them from how it really felt. I believe that real bravery comes from asking someone how they are and being fully prepared for whatever the answer is, even if it hurts you to hear it.

I didn't want to hurt my mum with my answer. I just wanted to be the brave one and get better and make her proud and move forward. I also got so used to just moving forward with my life that I never really took time to reflect on how having cancer affected me. Until it did.

'I don't care what anyone says, women have to know how to do everything in this world.'

That's what she would tell me – that I had to be independent. Well, now I am and I am starting my own family. As my brother and I grew up she just seemed to push us away. Or it felt like that. There were fights, and hurtful things were said. I don't know. It wasn't good.

Slowly we are working to repair our relationship. I never stopped loving her or sending her gifts. I just pulled away.

However, it's now Christmas Eve and I am suffering less from morning sickness and more from all-day sickness. I can't travel. I just can't face six hours on a bus. I'm pregnant and I can't drive – neither can Colm, but we're both arranging to get our provisional licences to start learning, at least.

I text my parents to tell them I am sick.

'Explosive diarrhoea,' I write.

I call them and ask to be put on speaker to both of them. Colm sits beside me.

'I'm not coming home for Christmas.'

My mother gets defensive, thinking it's an excuse and that I don't want to be there.

'I'm not coming home because . . . I'm pregnant.' I sob.

I cry because if you're raised Catholic, telling your parents you're pregnant is the worst thing possible, even if you're in your thirties and happily married.

They are shocked and delighted.

Then I tell them it's twins.

Swear words of delight erupt down the phone, my father jumping from happiness to not wanting to be happy in case his happiness jinxes it. Mum talks to me about how sick I am feeling and about taking care of myself. She sounds like my mum again. No defences, just worried about me, and I don't know how to feel.

25 December

We told Colm's family yesterday too. They're delighted we're spending Christmas in their house, literally up the road from ours, but I'm mostly upstairs away from the wonderfully nauseating yuletide yuck-smells.

28 December

My parents called to see me today. It's a big deal because, being from Donegal, my parents don't like to come to Dublin for any reason. It's as if the rest of the country hates Dublin and by going there it's somehow giving it attention and inflating its ego. I didn't think I'd end up living here, let alone marrying a Dubliner.

Colm and I have been together for years and usually it's us who go up to Donegal. My parents like him, mostly because he's a good man who makes me happy and isn't an arse.

When my parents see me they're shocked. I spent most of my life overweight, then the year I got married I decided to lose weight – not for the dress but for me. I lost 4 stone over two years, I think, but I'm tall so I can 'carry it'. However, the vomiting means I've lost weight I didn't intend to. My wedding ring fell off my finger on St Stephen's Night and I panicked looking for it. It turned up inside one of the big blankets under which I now live.

My parents hug me and tell me I'm too thin. They ask how Colm and I are, we talk about what's been going on and the conversation is good. We go for a carvery and I eat some food, then when we get back to the house I throw up again. Food just seems to shelter in my stomach rather than go anywhere productive. But overall this has been a good day.

1 January 2015

I rang in the New Year by eating crackers and drinking rehydration solution, just like in the movies. There aren't a lot of movies about pregnancy but there are so many movies about the actions that get you there. My god, if pregnancy were a movie it would be very dull, peppered with a lot of action scenes where someone is trying to find a toilet or a seat on a bus.

5 January

The majority of my text messages to Colm seem to be about how tired I am, how sick I feel and whether or not I've thrown up. I feel bad that I'm bombarding him with this level of detail but also feel that getting a play-by-

play is probably easier than actually going through it.
I tell him this.
He says, 'That's debatable.'

Week 11: Development

Your baby is as big as a (LIME)

This fact may remind you of Corona and the fact you can no longer drink or have ANY FUN!

Your baby has already chosen its favourite band but may change its mind many times during the pregnancy.

HOW YOU ARE FEELING

You ask loved ones IF YOU'VE GROWN FAT. Even if they say no, exclaim "I'm gonna get so FAT" in a sad whiney voice.

14 January

I have another bleed. I'm in work and I'm panicking because I have to leave but no one knows I'm pregnant yet, except John. I've no money for a taxi so he gives me a tenner and tells me that he'll cover for me. Colm says he will meet me at the hospital. I call my mum, who says it's probably nothing. Most of the time I try not to get attached to what is happening to me, in case something goes wrong, but then in moments like this I feel the devastation ready to crash into me. I am scanned, the twins are bigger and I'll be seen again next week for the 12 week scan. Apparently, bleeds just sometimes happen during the first trimester. For no apparent reason. Another fun symptom.

15 January

I've been reading a book about twins and decide to tell Colm what I've learned.

'Apparently, you shouldn't call them names which sound the same...'

'Like Lucas and Mucus?'

16 January

Today I told my boss that I am pregnant. It was incredibly difficult because there is no work-related opener for delivering that kind of news.

It feels as if I'm making a selfish choice that doesn't benefit my work or career because unfortunately my job isn't 'making babies'. If it was, I'm well above target with twins.

The reason I've been keeping it hidden from my work is to avoid letting people think that 'work isn't a priority for me, having a baby is.' And if I were to miscarry, then that information – that I want a baby – will be out there, and it will be out there for nothing.

THIS GRAPH REPRESENTS THIS WEEK'S DATA AND THE OTHER IS THE BABIES GROWING INSIDE ME

It's as if I can only focus on one thing or the other, or that I am choosing. Rather than being happy about it all, I just feel as if I'm letting my boss down and creating trouble. In contrast to this, Colm's boss was the first person he told, the week we found out. It turned out that his boss's wife was also pregnant.

Telling my co-workers was easier, mostly because some of them suspected and got to go 'I KNEW IT!'

Then I said, 'IN YOUR FACE, IT'S TWINS!'

The upside of telling people in work is, I guess, that I can vomit freely in the bathroom now without all the crazy subterfuge and feeling as if I'm in some sort of spy movie. Hopefully it won't change things with my colleagues, although we'll have to cancel Pâté Wednesdays, and Soft Cheese and Hair Dye Fridays.

19 January

We had the 12 week scan today. 'They're eleven weeks,' the sonographer said, and we found out that they are identical. I had a suspicion they were from my first scan, where my womb-mates just looked like peanuts exploring a cave. I only figured it out at 10 weeks, after googling scans for ages. I announced it to my husband, who was sceptical, but today I felt that warm fuzzy feeling of vindication, which was short-lived when they told me they were putting me on the MCDA protocol.

MCDA stands for monochorionic diamniotic. That is: one placenta but two sacs.

Twin pregnancies seem to work like this:

FRATERNAL TWINS (NON-IDENTICAL)

Two eggs, Two sperm!

two placentas
two amniotic
sacs.

IDENTICAL TWINS

←One egg, one sperm

← fertilized egg splits

placenta*

One or two amniotic sacs

* some identical twins can have two placentas depending on when the split occurs

Identical twins need to learn how to share from an incredibly young age. They share a placenta, which distributes blood and nutrients to each. Unfortunately, one twin can accidentally be a little too generous and pump too much away from itself and into the other. This is called twin-to-twin transfusion syndrome (TTTS) and puts both twins at risk. Because of this I have to be scanned every two weeks from 16 weeks.

Bloody hell, we're having identical twins.

25 January

Now that lots of people know I'm pregnant, I put it up on Facebook. Not with massive fanfare but using a photo of me beside a sign, outside an Italian restaurant I saw on the way back from Sweden, which said 'Prego'. Somewhere in the comments I put the fact it's twins. It feels as if all of this information at once would be a bit much, something I can't avoid when telling people in real life.

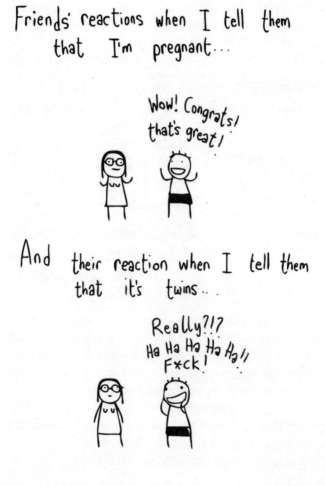

Friends' reactions when I tell them that I'm pregnant...

Wow! Congrats! that's great!

And their reaction when I tell them that it's twins...

Really?!? Ha Ha Ha Ha Ha!! F*ck!

SECOND TRIMESTER

2 February

Over coffee, Emma in work tells everyone that she is pregnant. It isn't twins. She said hearing me tell people the week before was surreal. She thought, 'What is happening? Am I saying this out loud?'

I'm happy for her. It is also really nice to have someone else going through this at the same time. Texting each other about pregnancy symptoms is reassuring and gives our husbands a break from it.

14 February

I made this card for Colm for Valentine's Day:

Roses are Red
Violets are Blue
Since you got me Pregnant
It's been difficult to Poo.
(But kinda worth it too)

15 February

My folks phoned. I told them I'm vomiting a lot this evening and still quite queasy. My mum mentions something about soup and I say, 'Don't talk about food.'

'I know you said not to talk about food,' Dad chimes in, 'but do you still like sushi?'

18 February

I'd been to Pilates before I fell pregnant. It was part of a cunning plan I'd had to stop my body from turning into a potato. I'd remembered my mother once saying, 'Pregnancy brings out any weakness your body has.' I guess she'd meant things such as old injuries rather than 'If you thought you had a problem with eating too many Big Macs before...'

If I'm honest, the real reason I'm going to carry on with it, but go to a special pregnancy class instead, is because my body already feels wrecked. Given the physical after-effects of cancer and the metal rod I have in my leg, it feels as if I need to do some damage limitation. I just want to get to the end of this pregnancy in one piece. Well, three pieces.

So yesterday I attended my first pregnancy Pilates class. The instructor went around the room and asked everyone how far along they were and how they were feeling. One woman was 39 weeks. I worried she'd give birth in the class and then wondered if I'd get a free class if she did.

'I'm sixteen weeks with twins,' I said when it was my turn. 'Still puking but have a bit more energy.'

Then she asked the girl next to me.

'I'm nineteen weeks. I hardly notice I'm pregnant at all!'

I didn't realize I could smother someone with a yoga mat.

Smother is as close to 'mother' as I feel right now.

28 February

So this evening my body decided, 'F**k it, let's make her look pregnant' – and this belly just appeared. I thought that it would be a gradual thing. Nope. Nope. Nope. Nope.

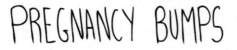

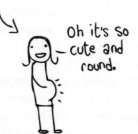

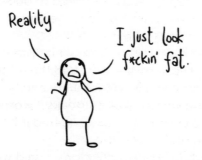

2 March

I've convinced Emma from work to go to pregnancy Pilates with me. So far my favourite part is when Rachel, the teacher, asks each person how they are doing and you get to, as briefly as possible, have a quick bitch about how being pregnant can be a bit crap and everyone nods.

9 March

Today I had my 18 week scan. It's fascinating to see the small peanuts becoming more human-looking. The sonographer talked at first, then went quiet. Then the silence spanned out until he said, 'I want to show this to someone else.'

He leaves then returns.

'When are you seeing the consultant?' he asks.

'In three weeks?'

'OK. I think you should see him today.'

One baby is smaller, it turns out, with less fluid around it.

The consultant's twin clinic didn't start until after 1 p.m., so Colm and I stood outside and I cried. I held Colm and I cried.

As exciting as getting scanned is, I was dreading any complications and now there are complications and we'd to wait until someone told us what they meant. We had tea and Colm read about Twin-to-Twin Syndrome and treatments, and he said it would be fine. I didn't want to read anything and create a disaster scenario in my head.

When we went back in to the hospital, we had to wait to see the consultant. We'd been warned in advance of his brusque and straight-to-the-point manner. Eventually we see him. He doesn't ask my name, shake my hand or introduce himself.

He takes the chart.

'You were scanned today?'

He measures my stomach with a tape measure.

'Everything looks fine. I'll see you in a month.'

'But . . . the size and the fluid? The guy who scanned me seemed concerned?'

'He's a little . . . inexperienced. Everything's fine. I don't want to see you again for a month.'

That was it. Two hours of worry resolved in two minutes of consultation.

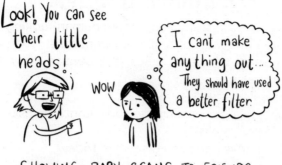

SHOWING BABY SCANS TO FRIENDS

12 March

Colm and I have been discussing baby names.

'Let's give one a normal name and the other a weird name!' I said.

'Like David...'

'...and Gandalf!'

Then I laughed at my own joke so much that I almost peed my pants outside Tesco.

15 March

Pregnancy sickness has been replaced by an ungodly hunger. Now I'm convinced that I'm having twins so that if I eat one I've a spare.

23 March

Today was the 20 week scan. We found out that they were girls. The handy thing about identical twins is you only need to see the genitals of one of them to tell.

I would have been happy either way, but when I told my mother she seemed disappointed.

'You thought they'd be boys?'

'Yes.'

PREGNANCY SYMPTOMS

If pregnancy were a medication, then the list of side effects would put off so many people. It felt as if every single thing that was happening to me – the vomiting, the drooling, the breathlessness, the large but sore breasts – was due to my pregnancy, and no one seemed very concerned.

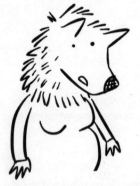

YES, YOU'VE TURNED INTO A WEREWOLF. THAT'S A NORMAL PREGNANCY SYMPTOM.

I would use the internet to look up every minor body change to make sure it was normal.

Google IS THIS NORMAL DURING PREGNANCY?

RESULTS

1. Woman asking the same question on a pregnancy forum...

2. Same as above, different forum.

3. Same thing again

I didn't want the paranoia of other pregnant women. Instead, I wanted the free internet advice of a medical professional.

I think back to when I was in my twenties and in my parents' kitchen with my brother. My mother is teasing us again about one of us having twins. My brother laughs but an image of identical twin girls flashes in my mind. Every time she teased us about it, that's what I saw. It never occurred to me that I could be having anything else.

25 March

I am 20 weeks pregnant. Every week I read updates on the babies' developmental progress – about what stage they are meant to be at. The Facebook of foetuses. There is a fruit and vegetable chart to go with this, to give me an idea of how big they are. They grow from the size of a poppy seed to a watermelon, which is impressive. More impressive is the fact that someone was able to come up with forty items of fruit and veg.

Where it falls down, if we're honest, is that a lot of fruits are the same size. A peach, a lemon and an orange, for example. However, every so often the chart would throw in a weirdly shaped fruit. This week the twins are each as big as a banana.

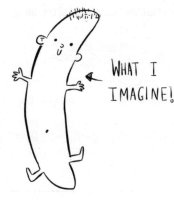

THIS WEEK YOUR BABY IS THE LENGTH OF A BANANA!

WHAT I IMAGINE!

27 March

Twenty-one weeks pregnant. Have succumbed to maternity jeans. They are very comfortable.

29 March

Colm and I are on a train, on our way to the Sunday market. There are two crying infants in our carriage. I look at Colm, then at my pregnant stomach, then at Colm again to see him mirroring my terrified expression.

31 March

Dietician: 'Your pregnancy weight gain is really good.'
Me: [*laughs in her face*]

8 April

I can feel the babies moving.

Rational brain: 'Babies moving, this is normal. They're moving. That's good. Normal. All perfectly normal.'

Irrational brain: 'THERE ARE TWO PEOPLE INSIDE ME HAVING A FECKING DANCE PARTY! WHAT IS HAPPENING?!'

14 April

Another week, another scan. Today it was the 24 week one.

I asked, 'What position are they in?'

The sonographer replied, 'Well, Twin A is head down, Twin B is head up. Look, Twin A's bum is in Twin B's face.'

'Wow, they've got a bit of a human centipede thing going on . . .'

Aside from that, the scan being OK means their risk of twin-to-twin transfusion syndrome goes way down, which is a relief.

We also saw one of them drinking the amniotic fluid – very cute. It became less cute when I later read that they wee into the amniotic fluid that they drink. Babies are weird.

17 April

Last night I was watching TV with my hands on my stomach, only to have them kicked from inside so hard that I screamed.

I have to keep reminding myself: 'It's all natural. It's not as weird as hell. They're not plotting against me.'

18 April

It was Emma's birthday, so I made her a card:

HAPPY BIRTHDAY

Treat yourself to

~~a glass of wine~~

~~Some soft cheese~~

~~a big piece of pâté~~

An iron supplement and a nap!

22 April

I farted during pregnancy Pilates. Then laughed.

To be fair, of all the things that could come out of you during pregnancy Pilates, a fart isn't the worst of them.

24 April

Someone gave me their seat on a packed bus. Genuinely delighted. Hooray for decent people!

25 April

Pregnancy goes on for longer than most TV series. (Unless we're including soap operas. And we aren't. There isn't a big enough cast and no soap opera is set in Cervix Close or Placenta Place.) It feels as if after the first episode, things plod along and nothing much happens. Sure, there are pockets of excitement along the way – enough to keep viewers interested. But generally things are a bit dull until the finale, and the finale is ages away.

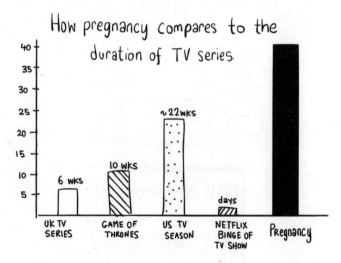

How pregnancy compares to the duration of TV series.

But for us, the finale was getting closer.

PREGNANCY FASHION

Pregnancy is one of the only human conditions that warrants its own fashion line. As much as you try to resist it, you end up succumbing at some stage.

I asked my friend Nina about bras.

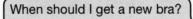

When should I get a new bra?

When you burst out of yours incredible hulk style in the middle of a meeting and milk drowns all your colleagues.

So I got a new bra.

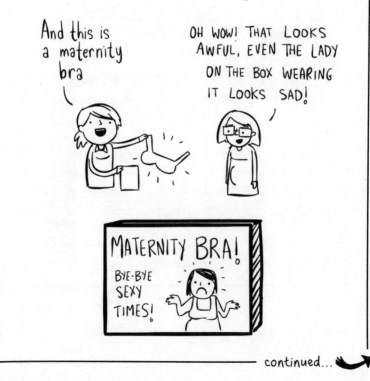

continued...

I thought pregnancy involved having a neat little bump to show that you're pregnant, but at the beginning it wasn't like that at all.

SCARF
- Hides developing preggie belly.
- Can be used to block out nausea-inducing smells.

STRIPY MATERNITY TOPS
- Nothing says "I'm Pregnant!" more than being huge and voluntarily choosing Horizontal stripes!

THE NON-MATERNITY COAT!
No one buys a new coat for this. Just wear your old coat until you can't close it. Then cover the exposed bits with a scarf.

Striped tops are such a popular maternity choice that when I was waiting in the hospital for my appointments, I would count how many women were wearing them. The highest number was seventeen; the lowest was three. Pregnancy is probably the only time I'll ever wear a piece of clothing that deliberately draws attention to my belly.

NAMING BABIES

Giving someone a name feels like a massive responsibility, a task Colm and I didn't take very seriously in the beginning.

The older you are when having children, the more individuals you will have met who have ruined perfectly good names. This is why more people are naming their kids weird stuff now.

'All the real names have been ruined, we're calling this child Cup-a-soup.'

To make things easier, I've developed a form, because nothing says responsible parenting like bureaucracy.

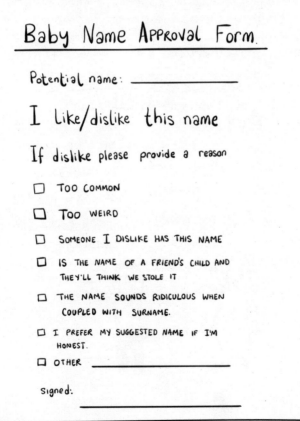

Baby Name Approval Form

Potential name: _____

I like/dislike this name

If dislike please provide a reason

☐ TOO COMMON

☐ TOO WEIRD

☐ SOMEONE I DISLIKE HAS THIS NAME

☐ IS THE NAME OF A FRIEND'S CHILD AND THEY'LL THINK WE STOLE IT

☐ THE NAME SOUNDS RIDICULOUS WHEN COUPLED WITH SURNAME.

☐ I PREFER MY SUGGESTED NAME IF I'M HONEST.

☐ OTHER _____

Signed:

_____

26 April

Yesterday, Colm and I attended an antenatal course run by the Irish Multiple Births Association. I was terrified beforehand, but it made me feel a bit better about having twins, mostly because someone there was expecting triplets.

So far I've treated pregnancy like a sickness, some bizarre, long-term medical condition which has meant I've spent a lot of time vomiting, my body has gone all weird, and I haven't really mentally engaged with the outcome. At the antenatal class, though, someone held a plastic baby and showed us how to bathe it. I've never bathed a baby. I've never even changed a nappy.

The reality of what is happening clicked in my head.

Last night, in the darkness of the bedroom, I started to cry.

'I'm scared,' I told Colm. 'I don't know how to deal with one baby, never mind two. Are you scared?'

'Yes, but I'm excited too.'

'What if I'm a bad mum? What if I can't do this?'

'We'll do it. It will be fine.'

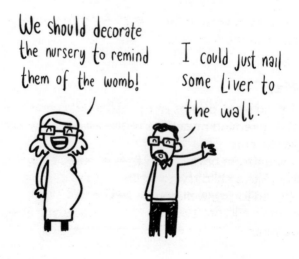

We should decorate the nursery to remind them of the womb!

I could just nail some liver to the wall.

THIRD TRIMESTER

12 May

Me: 'I have pregnancy asthma.'

Consultant: 'No, you have asthma which pregnancy has made a bit worse.'

I can't breathe as my growing children encroach on my lung space and try to escape through my mouth. I know their map-reading skills will improve and they will head south eventually. In the meantime, my GP wants to sign me off work. I cry. I say I can't, that I've too much to do.

And still I get bigger.

14 May

My bump feels hard. I'm asking people to touch it.

'Wow, it feels really hard.'

I do this because this may be the only time in my life someone will touch my belly and say that.

However, 'Wow, it feels really hard' got me into this situation in the first place. AMIRITE?!

16 May

I'm taking more photos of my expanding child farm. Mostly to remind myself down the line why my body looks like crap.

I went from having a small neat bump to basically looking like a child trying to dress up as Jupiter.

But seriously, well done boobs, for letting the side down and pretty much staying the same size throughout.

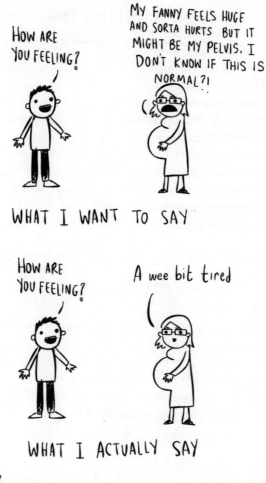

24 May

Colm and I went to IKEA today. I'm trying out armchairs – we don't have one at home. People say you need an armchair for breastfeeding; at the moment our seating options are a futon and a beanbag. I'm trying to find an armchair that I don't struggle to get out of.

There's another pregnant woman doing the same thing. We make eye contact and I smile at her.

She doesn't acknowledge me.

She hurries away.

Something I've noticed about pregnant women is that very often we actively ignore one another. Once I saw it happening, I wanted to understand why.

A fun fact about pregnant women: they avoid other pregnant women like the plague because they want to feel special. If, as a fellow preggo, you break that rule and actually look or smile at them, they don't know how to deal with it. You've taken away their feeling of being special.

For this reason I love following pregnant women around IKEA.

Rubbing my big belly.

NOT SO SPECIAL NOW, ARE YOU?!

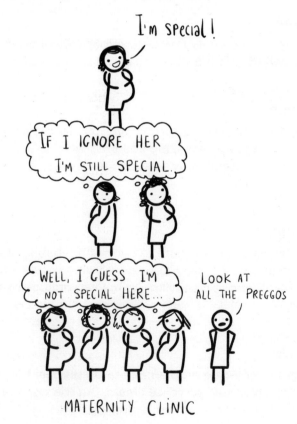

25 May

I sneezed loudly, then said, 'F**k's sake.'

Colm said, 'A bit of wee came out, didn't it?'

He wasn't wrong.

26 May

I am tired and big, and the consultant has written me a letter saying I need to stop working. He doesn't even know my name; he started my maternity letter with, 'This lady...'

I find that somewhat endearing.

8 June

First day of maternity leave. Have found that I can fill large periods of time worrying about the future.

12 June

Going to a wedding tomorrow. Got my hair cut and my eyebrows done. Still feel big and pregnant.

This is probably how a balloon feels when you draw a face on it.

17 June

I just farted so loudly that I felt one of the babies startle inside me.

The other one clearly knows me well enough by this stage.

20 June

I've got ninety-nine problems because pregnant women aren't allowed soft-serve ice cream. But the weather's so hot. It's hot and everything is swelling.

When I had my cancer removed at fifteen, they took some of the lymph nodes in my groin with it. This means that my right leg swells generally – something I'm not delighted with, but if that's the price I pay to be alive...

My mother's warning that 'pregnancy brings out any weakness your body has' has come to pass. So I've carried on with the pregnancy Pilates – not just the classes but every night at home – and have been rubbing oil over my expanding belly as if I'm basting myself ready for the oven. So much work just to stop my body from crumbling under the strain of it all.

21 June

Colm spent some of Father's Day washing baby clothes.

Meanwhile, his children are completely unaware that Father's Day exists or that they'll even need clothes.

23 June

Thirty-four weeks pregnant.

Went for another scan. The twins now weigh 5lbs each. This is good because I said I'd be happy to get them over 5lbs, and now here we are.

The consultant said, 'I'll see you in three weeks!'

'But I thought I was giving birth in two weeks, when I'm thirty-six weeks?'

'Thirty-seven weeks is time enough.'

I told him I wanted a C-section, I'd decided it. He tried to talk me out of it: did I realize I could always try to push them out myself? I hadn't even considered that was an option and it came as a bit of a shock. Afterwards, I felt a bit tearful. Firstly, they're big babies – 10lbs in total right now – and I've three more weeks, and secondly, I'm thinking I might actually try to push them out myself.

Lots to think about, or avoid thinking about.

I messaged my mother-in-law.

> Asked if I'm getting a
> c-section, he said 50/50.
> Which scared me. 15:07 ✔✔

> Don't be scared. It's another
> form of birth. By the due date
> you won't care if they take
> babies out through your ear.
> 15:11

> Ha ha ha! 15:18 ✔✔

24 June

So I found out that my dad has colon cancer. He'd sent away a sample to be screened, it came back positive, they gave him a colonoscopy and they found the cancer. He had no notable symptoms.

Perhaps having had cancer myself made me more pragmatic about the news. I saw the results of the colonoscopy as a bit like someone telling you your laces are undone before you trip. But it's cancer. I think my honest reaction was, 'This is good, it's been caught early.'

Often, people don't want to talk about an illness such as cancer because they feel that even saying the word is inviting it into their lives. I wasn't hugely worried, though. I asked my parents what the staging of the cancer was, went off to read about it and what would happen next, then relayed back to them the information I'd found.

I then bought Dad a Father's Day card that says 'Dad, You're a Bad Ass!'

It's funny because it's cancer.

27 June

My body is finally starting to crumble under the weight of carrying twins. Hip pain I've been feeling for the past few days has worsened to the point where walking is hard and crying is easier.

I booked an appointment with a physio at short notice. Fifteen minutes' notice...When I got there she asked how pregnant I was.

'Almost thirty-five weeks with twins.'

'OK, I need you to loosen your clothes.'

'Actually, I need to take off this pelvic support first...'

I lifted my shirt to take off the support and she exclaimed, 'Wow, you're really big!'

After people telling me for ages, 'You're really small for twins,' 'You're really neat,' 'You wouldn't know it was twins,' this was the first time someone had called me big, knowing I'm carrying two babies. To be honest, it was a relief.

Then she massaged my hip and back for half an hour as I flinched and cried, but it was worth it.

'All the pain is muscular. The muscles are all really tight.'

Except my pelvic floor, obviously, as I'm still treating every sneeze as a threat.

Three more weeks of this crap.

Three more weeks.

1 July

My dad requested to have his operation in Dublin – to be closer to me – and my mother ended up staying with me and Colm. My aunt is stopping over at my parents' house to keep an eye on my sister, as although she has a level of independence, she can't be left on her own overnight.

'Wow, your belly has dropped a lot,' Mum said when she saw me. 'You could give birth any day now.'

Now I'm paranoid that I'm giving birth any day now. Thanks, Mum.

2 July

My dad is going into hospital to have the cancer in his colon removed this morning.

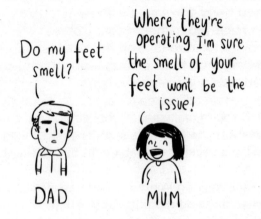

3 July

The last few weeks of pregnancy seem to involve my body being tortured until I say, 'I'm ready to be a parent, make this stop, please!'

Feeling cumbersome and big, all of the strength I put into doing Pilates and working out the whole time I've been pregnant has got me as far as this week. Now, my right hip no longer thinks it should support me in this endeavour. From a resting position, the first few steps are the hardest as I'm unsure whether my right leg will actually move, but once I get going it isn't so bad. Just...awkward.

I'm ready for this parenthood thing, and I'm not. I'm elated at the idea of giving birth and frightened at the same time. How did we suddenly end up here?

The bump is now huge, though people still say I'm neat. As if because I'm carrying twins, my stomach is meant to resemble something from the end of *Ghostbusters*. I am the Stay Puft Marshmallow Man: enormous, marching through the city, angry and afraid. I'm pretty sure he never wanted to be that big or to explode into a sticky mess.

I will miss the bump. I will miss touching my stomach unashamedly and drawing attention to it – something I never did in the past. I'm the kind of person who hides it behind a cushion when I sit down but now, look at me, it's huge. I don't care.

Rubbing it, I feel the babies move. Twin A, or CoJu, is motivated mostly by food – the idea that I'm eating – and Twin B, or MaJu, is quieter.

We've found that MaJu likes some music. Lying in bed, holding a speaker near her and playing 'Martha' by Tom Waits, she moves. Either she really loves the song or she's afraid of Tom Waits.

Colm declares it time for a 'baby inspection' if I say they're moving. He holds his hand against my stomach and says, 'Hmm-hmm, hmm-hmm, yes, there are babies in there' with a certainty that only a qualified baby inspector would have.

I'll miss this – these wrigglers who are trying to destroy my body with their occupancy. In a week or so it will be over. I can put a hand on to them now and feel their backs, maybe a shoulder (actually, I've no idea). The one thing I do know is that when one of them (CoJu) hiccups, I feel it against my asshole. This is not a welcome feeling.

I already miss their movements, that is until I get up and try to walk, then I think it's probably a good idea that they come out.

Another week or so of this, another week or so of MaJu and CoJu. After that, we'll see. Something good, I hope. Another adventure.

4 July

When Colm's in the sitting room, I've started entering bump-first, allowing it to appear slowly from behind the door as I hum the theme tune to *2001: A Space Odyssey*.

5 July

Went to see Dad in hospital. Gave him a get well soon card. On the inside I wrote, 'Congrats on your poo!'

He had a poo. That's good news. Also, today is the first day I haven't accidentally seen his balls since he was admitted.

thumbs up

6 July

Saw Dad in hospital again. Things have gone from 'his bowel is working' to 'his bowel is working too well'. He's gone from projectile vomiting *Exorcist*-style to being afraid to fart. He's not really eating yet, so everything is water and bile and trying to convince him to drink something.

The thing is, in that hospital I see a sicker, weaker version of the man I know. More quiet and tired, and at times a bit confused, but still my dad. To me, he's not an old man, he's a strong man; a man who wants to know who you are and where you're from in case he knows your neighbours.

7 July

Saw my consultant; I'm booked in for induction next Wednesday. Though he said I might give birth before then.

The end is in sight.

I've never been more terrified or excited.

8 July

Dad has been discharged from hospital into the care of my mother. He says repeatedly that he regrets the operation, that he wasn't sick, and now he feels destroyed. I tell him I understand, because I do, more than anyone, and I tell him that I want him to be around to see his granddaughters. Because I think that they'll really like him.

9 July

Less than a week of pregnancy left and the physio has given me a crutch to help me walk. It turns out that a twin pregnancy and pre-existing problems from cancer surgery don't mix. Although at least this time I get to take the growths home with me and put clothes on them and for it not to be 'weird'.

I told my friend John that I'd been given a crutch.

> I got a crutch today to help me walk. Super sexy

> Now you can fulfil your life long dream of being a mobile pole dancer

> Ha ha ha ha

14 July

Today is my last day of pregnancy.

I never thought I'd make it here, to 37 weeks, to having twins, who are technically full term (the last few weeks of pregnancy after this would be 'fattening them up').

Today I have a bump and I'm full of babies and all the emotion that tomorrow, things change.

I pause while writing this and rub the bump anxiously, realizing that I've been doing so for the past few weeks as a comfort, to them and myself. As excited as I am about no longer being pregnant and about getting my body back from the hostage stand-off that has been escalating for the last month or two, I am, at this moment, afraid.

Up to this point pregnancy has been a condition. Sure, at the back of my mind I knew that I'd have to give birth and that there would be babies, but in amongst the side effects and troubles, that moment was far ahead in the future. Now, suddenly, it's not. I'm afraid because I've never done this before. I know that lots of women go through it and they're fine, and people tell me it will be fine, but there's a lot of 'what if it's not' whirring around at the back of my mind.

Pregnancy was/is lonely.

Pregnancy swallows your body, your mind, your freedom, your wardrobe and your conversation. You don't mean for that to happen but it does. And you want to talk about it but you're sick of talking about it, and people will say they understand what you're going through but you are, for the most part, going through it alone. I don't mean to say that people aren't great about it, because they are, and it's nice to hear kind words and know that you're not going crazy. But I doubt that anyone else is thinking about my pregnancy as much as I am, because frankly, I can't get away from it.

Except that tomorrow I can.

After tomorrow I'll no longer be the person declaring to her husband that she is an egg, then chanting, 'Egg! Egg! Egg!' while wandering the house rubbing her belly or giving him a blow-by-blow account of what his giant children are doing to her insides.

Tomorrow, he becomes a father, I become a mother and they become people I cannot foresee.

But at this moment in time, I am still pregnant.

I am excited.

I am afraid.

I will be fine.

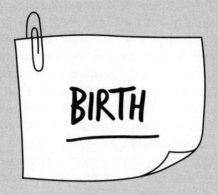

Before I gave birth, I'd been going to Pilates, had taken an antenatal class and had been listening to a hypnobirthing album at night. I first heard hypnobirthing affirmations when I tried acupuncture for pregnancy nausea (which didn't work). The therapist played a track to me while I still had needles in my body. As I lay there listening to a woman telling me that everything was going to be fine, and saying something like, 'Your body is ready for your baby', I laughed so incredibly hard that the needles came out of my ears.

As my due date approached, however, I turned to those affirmations in desperation. I was having trouble sleeping because I was massive and felt a constant urge to pee – an annoyance compounded by the fact that our only toilet was downstairs at the other end of the house. So when I couldn't sleep and found myself lying awake and worrying, I would put on the hypnobirthing CD because the lady on it was the only one who was going to reassure me at 4 a.m. that everything was going to be fine. She said I could do this, she said I would be fine, she also kept saying 'baby' and not 'babies' because she didn't know.

She was trying to prepare me for giving birth but I didn't really feel prepared, I felt I was letting her down.

At the antenatal class we were advised to draw up a birth plan. At that point I thought I was having a C-section. Then, when both babies were head down I was persuaded to push them out the 'in-door'. What changed after that was this: CoJu was head down, but MaJu was head up. I was still given the OK to push but our birth plan became this:

BIRTH PLAN
* Get these babies out of *
me safely!
please.

Giving birth is a lot like doing your Leaving Cert: there's a huge build-up and people like to tell you exactly how they did, but after a few years it doesn't matter. Much like your exam results, there aren't many opportunities in everyday life to actually talk about how you gave birth. It's not like showing someone a cake and telling them the recipe.

While I was still pregnant I found that expectant mums are a good excuse for other mothers to relay their birth stories – in the same way someone might tell a spooky story around a campfire. However, if I'm honest, I didn't really pay attention to the tales I heard because I literally had no context for what I was being told. It's all well and good saying, 'It's like squeezing a melon out something the size of a lemon,' but that's not a sensation. You might as well tell the baby that being born is like trying to get their head through the neck

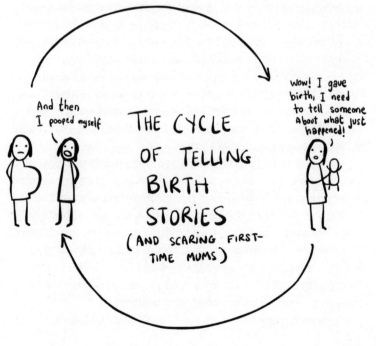

And then I pooped myself

THE CYCLE OF TELLING BIRTH STORIES (AND SCARING FIRST-TIME MUMS)

Wow! I gave birth, I need to tell someone about what just happened!

of a jumper that is way too small, because they have no idea what a jumper is.

What I've realized is that childbirth is like losing your virginity: the end result is the same but everyone's story about the event itself is different. I went into giving birth the way I go into most things in life: fairly clueless but willing to give it my best shot.

MY BIRTHING STORY, WHERE I MANAGED NOT TO POOP MYSELF

When I was 37+1, I was told I'd be giving birth to my twins by hook or by crook. Turns out they literally meant by hook, as I had my waters broken at about ten in the morning on 15 July. My Pilates teacher, Rachel, had told us that when waters break it doesn't happen like it does in the movies – it's not this big flood of liquid, apparently. Well, in my case, it was as if my labour had been directed by Michael Bay: my waters absolutely poured out of me. So much so that the midwife actually made a note that it was a lot, then kept telling the other midwives it was a lot. All while I'm standing there like something you'd see in Yellowstone National Park.

After that they wanted to see if my contractions would start naturally, which involved me fannying around on an exercise ball for two hours. It wasn't enough so I was given an oxytocin drip and then, an hour later, an epidural and Colm was told to deflate the ball he'd spent five minutes inflating. Initially the epidural made my blood pressure crash so rapidly I passed out, but after that there was a lot of waiting around, lying on a bed having the twins monitored, just waiting.

I have to say, the staff were amazing during all

this. I spent the whole day in the birthing suite being monitored, and after a lot of oxytocin and contractions I got to 10cm dilated at half past midnight. I can't lie, I was knackered and the pushing part hadn't even started.

'OK, we're going to get you to push now.'

'What do I do?'

'Push against your bum.'

It turns out that labour is a lot like pregnancy Pilates. I had a nice woman telling me to use muscles beyond what was comfortable, for longer than was comfortable, and it involved a lot of breathing. Although pregnancy Pilates does require that you wear pants and no one puts their hand up you during plank.

At one point in the labour, my temperature went up to 38°C and MaJu started to become distressed.

'We need to cut you to help this along. Is that OK?'

I said yes. If I'd been told, 'We need to feed you fifty hot dogs to help this along' I would have said, 'That's a bit unconventional, but sure.' I just wanted the twins to be OK. After CoJu came out, she was handed to Colm, who held her against his bare chest, like they were a poster from the 1990s.

I had to prepare for round two, but I was still worried about MaJu. She'd been presenting breech before I went into labour. The doctors warned me that if she stayed that way it would be fine, but if she moved in some weird position I'd need a C-section, and I was OK with that. They're scanning me, trying to see her position and I'm nervous and worried. Then they say it: she's flipped spontaneously to a head-down position, the little beauty. She was born with much less effort (my fanny basically a swing door by this stage) twelve minutes after her sister.

Now they were in the world, they were no longer CoJu and MaJu. We named them alphabetically in order of appearance: Bronagh and Róisín. They weighed 5lbs 14oz and 5lbs 10oz.

They were out; they were healthy.

Months later, in conversation, people would assume I had a Caesarean. I'd correct them, tell them I pushed out both babies and make them give me a high five, but in the long term it doesn't really matter. All birth is natural birth.

THIS BABY
CAME OUTTA ME!

NATURAL BIRTH

BABY I
SUMMON THEE

SUPERNATURAL BIRTH

Both babies were born with their eyes wide open, staring at us – at everyone – trying to figure out what had just happened. And we stared right back, in the shock and awe that comes with suddenly having two babies. One of the doctors gave me Róisín to hold; it felt really surreal to do so after all this time.

Why giving birth is a bit like 😊 meeting someone from the Internet

1. You've known them by a nickname and it feels weird to call them by their real name.

2. They look nothing like their picture.

3. It's usually a good idea not to meet them on your own.

In movies I'd seen women in full make-up give birth after two decent pushes. They held their babies and everyone cried for joy. It wasn't like that for me. The birth plan of 'evacuate all personnel from my body safely' had worked. I was happy but I was mostly relieved. Then the reality hit us: we had two babies.

'We have two babies,' I said to Colm.

'I know,' he replied. 'There are two babies who were inside you, but now they are here.'

I thought that someone might demonstrate how babies worked, and when I'd shown some competency in the role of mother I'd be given full responsibility for them.

But the responsibility was immediate.

'Here are your babies.'

They thought I knew what I was doing. I didn't. But I was going to learn.

NEWBORNS

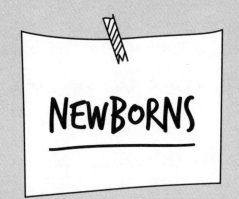

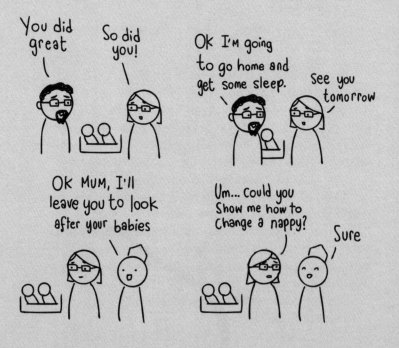

Why being with a newborn baby in hospital is like being at a music festival. ♫

1. You get a wristband.

2. You don't get much sleep.

3. You're dying for a shower.

4. IT GETS REALLY LOUD!

5. IT's messier than you imagined

6. You can get your boobs out and no one bats an eyelid.

7. You can't wait to get home to your own bed.

As an introduction to being a parent, having twins is like buying a video game you've never played before and saying, 'I'll start it on EXPERT.'

I fully intended to breastfeed them and after they were born the midwife managed to get them both to latch on to me. Nothing quite prepared me for the surreal nature of that. One of the bodily changes I was most alarmed by in late pregnancy was my boobs gearing themselves up to BE FUNCTIONAL. Each one felt like an evolving Pokémon reaching their final and true form.

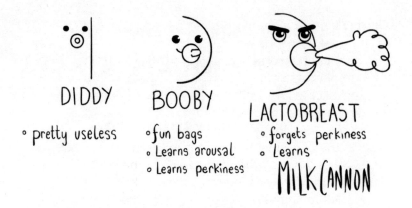

DIDDY
◦ pretty useless

BOOBY
◦ fun bags
◦ Learns arousal
◦ Learns perkiness

LACTOBREAST
◦ forgets perkiness
◦ Learns

MILK CANNON

If I'm honest, I thought that breastfeeding a baby would be fairly straightforward: they find the nipple and they suck it, and milk comes out because that makes sense. But it wasn't. There was this whole latching thing, where a baby has to be attached properly in order for the breast to release milk. The closest thing I can imagine it being like is a spaceship docking: the airlock can't be opened unless the spaceship is docked correctly. None of us had ever been to space before.

Feeding was difficult. One of the twins was better than the other at latching; the other would get frustrated with my boob and end up head-butting it. I tried to express milk myself and used a syringe to feed them. When one of their blood sugars dipped, a midwife suggested I top them up with formula. I did.

I was immediately given the basic instructions that I had to change, feed and settle two newborn babies every three hours, and in the beginning the task took almost two and a half hours to complete. At night, one twin would wake, look at me and then cry, and I'd hold her, hoping that the other didn't wake up, because I was finding handling one newborn baby challenging enough, their warm body against mine, in the small quiet moments before the feeding cycle started again.

Even though I was sharing my room at the hospital

with two other women and their babies, I felt very alone, as if I were someone drafted in to boost morale.

'It could be worse, I could be yer wan with the twins.'

I remember sitting up in bed in a near-dark room at 4 a.m., just me and whichever baby I happened to be feeding and trying to keep them quiet as everyone else in the room slept.

On the plus side, I'd got to grips with nappy changes. The babies, on the other hand, hadn't. They didn't understand why I was intermittently making them cold. They took me removing their nappy as their cue to wee everywhere. Either that or they were busy making their first poops, which seemed to be made of treacle from hell.

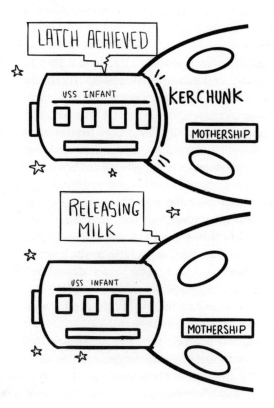

17 July

Text message to Colm:

> Just a heads up. I've had a hour of sleep. Maybe hour and a half.
> 09:00 ✓✓

> Long night of feeding?
> 09:03

> Feeding, puking, pooping, crying and that was just me.
> 09:05 ✓✓

18 July

Last night involved one hour of sleep again, before a midwife stepped in and took one of the babies to be fed. She told me to sleep, and when she popped back I was weeping silently. She said it was exhaustion and hormones. She was nice, and very matter of fact with the babies, affectionately calling them maggots.

She'd responded to a call bell from me at 4 a.m. I'd been standing, holding one twin because she was upset and wanted to be held, only to have the other realize what an amazing plan that was and she now wanted in on the action. It felt like that scenario with the boatman and the chicken, the fox and the grain. Except the boatman had only had three hours' sleep in two days and needed a bigger boat.

In that moment the whole thing felt overwhelming.

I'm certain I will feel that again.

The babies are now less like small bodily-fluid-making machines; their other desires are kicking in, apparently at three in the morning. Róisín looked at me and there was something in the way she did so that said,

'I know you, you're the warm boob thing.' Not a loving look; more calculated. I'm being played.

The doctors wanted to keep me in hospital for a third day, but I couldn't stay any longer. It wasn't because of the babies that I wasn't sleeping, it was because the other women in the room were talking on their phones during the time I could be sleeping. I felt like I was going insane. If I was at home, at least Colm could help me.

So today I went home to be with my new family and actually rest in a bedroom that doesn't have two women chatting on their phones from 10 p.m. until after 2 a.m. Thankfully, the only mobile the babies have involves animals slowly revolving to the sounds of Bach.

I cried in front of the lift when they said I could leave the hospital, then again outside the hospital when we were leaving, then again when I saw the twins at home in their little cot.

Meanwhile, the cat knows something is going on and is eyeing me with suspicion.

19 July

My mum and dad came to Dublin yesterday to help and to stay overnight. My dad is still recovering from his surgery and is tired but trying to help. I, on the other hand, have reached the point of exhaustion where I have started to hallucinate. But now I've had four hours' sleep, as much as I've had since they were born.

Before I became a mum, I had never held a newborn baby. I think newborns are for the 'I really like babies' kind of people – people who've either held a baby before or are way more confident in their ability not to drop one than I was. I had never even seen a baby up close like this, so small and delicate.

Newborns will try to distract you from their

MY DAD

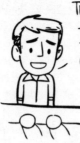

They are amazing.
I'm so proud of you.
You did brilliant!

ALSO MY DAD

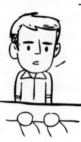

That one looks hungry, would ya not give her a bit of an egg?

They were four days old

weakness through one display of strength: they will, if you offer them your finger or thumb, grip it and try to crush it with their tiny hand. They are born with an invaluable social gift: the ability to give a firm handshake. And they hope that as a first impression it's enough for you to forgive the second impression they might make. It sort of worked – whenever I think about my babies that image flashes in my head: an impossibly small and perfectly formed hand wrapped around my finger, trying to pulverize it.

If life is a party, then the first thing we invite babies to do when they enter the world is to make the loudest

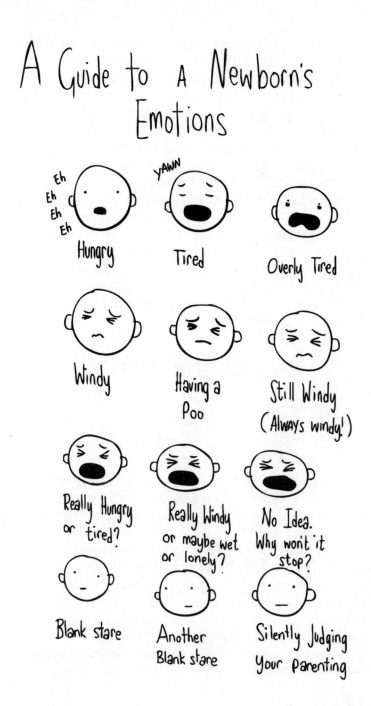

noise they can to let everyone know that they've arrived. That first cry inflates their lungs but what's more impressive is how loud it can be. In terms of 'loudness', normal speech is 60dB but the most frequent new-parent conversations occur at a whisper (20dB).

A baby's cry, however – that's loud. It's really loud, but it isn't as loud as say a jackhammer (100dB). No, it's louder. Babies cry at around 110dB, which is the average pain threshold for sound. I found out this information from a scientific paper that suggested that people who work regularly with babies should wear earplugs, as they might do at a rock concert. And after I heard the cry once, I seemed to spend most of my time avoiding hearing it again. Unfortunately for me, the cry seems to be the favoured means of communication for newborns' needs, all of which are extremely important and require attention immediately.

Why is the baby crying?

Wet? ☐
Cold? ☐
Warm? ☐
Hungry? ☐
Tired? ☐
Lonely? ☐

It's figured out that I don't really know what I'm doing? ☐

When I couldn't figure out what was the matter, holding a baby as she cried, a small voice in my head would whisper quietly:

When both of the babies cried at the same time we called it the 'Doomsday scenario'.

23 July

The twins are a week old today.

'Good work. You've done great! You're a great dad,' I told Colm.

'I'm working on different "dad phases",' he replied. 'This week "great dad", then next week "absent dad" where I go out for milk and come back a week later, with a tan and some postcards from Spain.'

24 July

After a week or so, I am starting to feel that maybe I'm getting better at looking after them. The house contains the babies and the people who are willing to care for them but it also contains all of the things that we need to keep our newborn overlords contented. And, like a scientist happy to do experiments within the confines of a laboratory, I am not confident in my abilities in the real world. My anxiety about being a new parent is in direct correlation to the distance I am from the confines of our home. And because neither of us can drive yet (although Colm has been learning for a good few months) we have to bring the twins in the buggy anywhere we go.

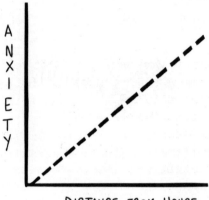

DISTANCE FROM HOUSE

28 July

Today we brought the babies on a bus to a shopping centre. All Colm's idea, as my tendency to disasterize everything means that given the choice, I would put off any kind of excursion until they turn eighteen. It would be just us, shut in a house, slowly going mad because I worry I can't cope outside with two babies.

The trip went fine, although I was incredibly anxious for some of the time – an immense, suffocating anxiety that made me want to cry and escape back home as quickly as possible in case I couldn't cope and I'm doing this all wrong. Then there's the guilt that I don't want the twins to have this anxiety-riddled mother who doesn't want to show them the world because she's afraid that she can't.

Tomorrow Colm, the calmer of us, goes back to work and it will be just me, two babies and a cat. I worried about that too, in between worrying about everything else.

I can do this.
I'm doing OK.
I'm not f**king it up.
At least that's what my mantra will be tomorrow.

29 July

Colm went back to work and I got a visit from the public health nurse. She was nice enough but I felt as if I was a bit like a box for her to tick.

'Are you feeding them yourself?'

'I'm combi-feeding but they're mostly getting formula.'

'I'm going to put down that you're breastfeeding.'

Then she weighs them.

'Your babies have gained weight. Well done, Mum!'

Healthcare workers congratulate you on successfully fattening your offspring.

Unfortunately I love praise, so I keep feeding them up and I keep getting praise. Then there's a tipping point: the babies are huge, the healthcare worker purses her lips.

'No, this is too much weight.'

But it's too late.

They eat the healthcare worker.

1 August

On 1 August 1996 I had my operation to remove the cancer from my lymph nodes. It was malignant melanoma, a statistical anomaly, a fluke of cell division for the cancer to have evolved from an existing mole in someone so young.

I take 1 August as the anniversary of getting rid of the cancer because it's easy to remember but also difficult to forget. I don't celebrate it openly because that somehow feels gleeful, so when we realized that

Colm first grew a beard in 1996 we celebrate that instead. So today is 'nineteen years of beard'.

Nineteen years have passed, and in a way none have.

I find myself inexplicably mother to identical twin girls.

They are a statistical anomaly, a fluke of cell division.

The only cancer afflicting them is their star sign.

5 August

Most nights after 5 p.m. the babies cry intensely for a period of time. Some people call this the witching hour, which is a lie as it lasts for more than an hour. We call these episodes 'Vietnam flashbacks' because the twins cry so fiercely, with a look on their faces as if they're remembering some horror they've witnessed.

I go into the spare room, holding whichever one of them is the worst affected. I sit on the pile of clothes that is covering the bed and tell them it will be OK, even though they don't understand what I'm saying. Even though I don't either.

10 August

I am spending time on my own with the babies, waiting for Colm to come home. It is always very busy with the washing, the feeding, the nappy changes . . . The first day Colm went back to work he thought I was going to sit down, watch Netflix and relax. I laughed really loudly at him, the intensely high-pitched laugh of 'I HAVE NEVER HEARD ANYTHING MORE RIDICULOUS!'

13 August

After the kids were born we got so many wonderful cards, presents and well-wishes from friends and family. Family I hadn't talked to in years, all welcoming our children into the world. It was wonderful and touching that they cared so much about this big event in our lives.

My extended family is big – my parents are both from families with seven kids, and Colm and I are both from families with three. Colm is the middle child. His older brother lives in London and his other brother is seven years younger and at an age where babies are a terrifying unknown. Some of Colm's confidence with babies comes from having a younger brother.

I, on the other hand, don't have a younger sibling – I'm the youngest. My mother always liked to introduce me as 'my baby'. I say 'liked to' but she still does it. Complications during my birth resulted in her needing 14 units of blood, dying on the table twice, and eventually, to stop the bleeding, they gave her a hysterectomy. That's why I'm the youngest. She said she didn't see me for five days after I was born, and when I ask her what her first impression of me was, she says, 'You smelled of curry.'

As well as my brother who lives in Sweden and is two years older, I also have a sister who is four years older. When she was very young, my sister didn't speak. They tested her hearing and she wasn't deaf. She is autistic and moves between two worlds – hers and ours. When she was younger she spent so much time in her own world that, to be safe there, our world had to be regimented and predictable, so she would be undisturbed by it. The rocking motions, the staring into space, the rhythms of things soothed her – they all made her feel secure.

Over the years she moved more into our world. Her mood calmed, and there was no more rocking, though she still becomes anxious at massive and unpredictable changes. Although she's able to go to the shops, live her life well in my parents' small town and people are nice to her, she can't be left on her own overnight. That's why, when my parents come up to Dublin, they usually have to go back within the day, though sometimes one of my aunts will stay over and mind her so they can stay away for longer.

Colm's parents have been running a launderette for years. It's a place full of bags of clothes and mountains of ironing – my personal hell. They are trying to wind it down and move outside of Dublin. They are busy and I know they feel bad that they aren't around more. But Colm and I have each other.

Having babies has transformed our relationship. Firstly, we combined our genetic material into two entirely new people, and secondly, we're going to look after them until some distant point in the future when they'll be able to look after themselves but still come back home with a bag of dirty laundry.

Looking after babies is hard work – not just all of the activities involved in order to silence the 'something is wrong' crying, but all the activities that support those activities. Colm is still my husband whom I love very much, but he's also become my co-worker in the business of baby-wrangling, which seems to be a 24-hour business.

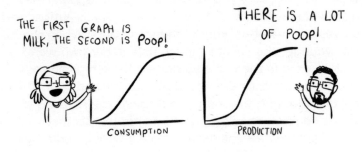

15 August

Having babies is odd. If they're upset, I whip out my boobs. I can't do that in other aspects of my life.

'I'm sorry for your loss . . .'

lifts top

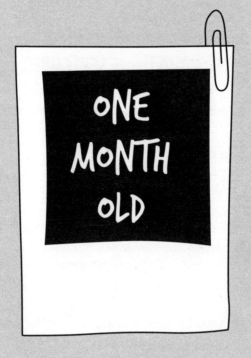

16 AUGUST - 15 SEPTEMBER

* Makes eye contact and stares at faces

* Responds to parent's voice

* Lifts head while lying on tummy

* Moves head from side to side while lying on tummy

* Follows objects briefly with eyes

* Begins to coo, gurgle and make other vocal sounds

* Makes equal movements with hands and feet

16 August

Week one: 'We're not going to give them soothers for ages.'
Week four: 'Quick! Go out and buy more soothers before the shop shuts!'

17 August

Babies decimate your life. It's as if they take everything you could conceive as being part of a normal adult existence and cast it into the fire of responsibility. For the first few weeks it is all about the babies because that is how they engineer it.

Want to eat some food? Well, you can't because the babies are crying. They want *their* food. You must give them their food. Your food must wait. So you feed them, willing them to eat faster, before spending what feels like the next two hours trying to get them to burp. Then it's time to feed them again. Your food must wait.

Do you know what tastes better the more you microwave it? Nothing. Nothing tastes good after it's been reheated four times. Colm and I survived mostly on toast and sandwiches in the early weeks, and a few times we got pizza delivered. Basically, we ate any food you can devour quickly with one hand because the other is occupied by a child. Sure, you could use a fork to eat a warm meal, but do you trust yourself not to spill hot food on your child's head? Just kidding, there's no chance the food would still be hot by the time you got to it.

19 August

The babies are feeding fine. Although I don't have a reference point for that other than the fact that they are gaining weight. One month down the line I am still trying to combi-feed, which basically involves trying

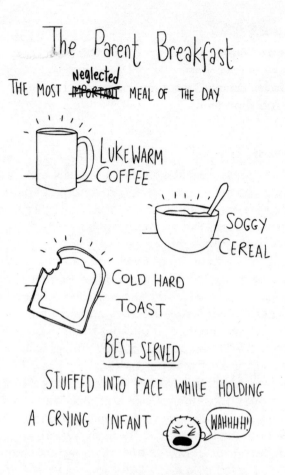

The Parent Breakfast

THE MOST ~~IMPORTANT~~ neglected MEAL OF THE DAY

LUKEWARM COFFEE

SOGGY CEREAL

COLD HARD TOAST

BEST SERVED

STUFFED INTO FACE WHILE HOLDING A CRYING INFANT

WAHHHH!

to breastfeed/express milk/sterilize bottles/make up formula. Sometimes the twins spit up after they've fed. In an attempt to help with this, we've changed their type of bottle. Our thought process as we browsed the various ranges was: 'What bottle can we use that won't turn these babies into a formula fountain?' Unfortunately, the bottles we settled on have seven parts to them and have to be disassembled, cleaned, sterilized and reassembled before being loaded with milk.

It's a lot of work – like doing *The Crystal Maze*, but every zone is 'the Parenting Zone' – and with two babies feeding every three hours, my hands are as dry as the feet of a budgie from washing them all the time. On top of this, I'm also trying to breastfeed or express milk from my now functional boobs, which are not producing a lot of milk but are giving it a go.

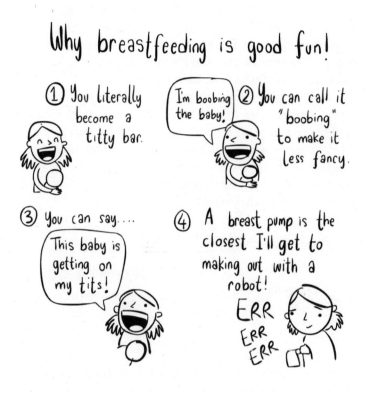

Why breastfeeding is good fun!

① You literally become a titty bar.

I'm boobing the baby!

② You can call it "boobing" to make it less fancy.

③ You can say....

This baby is getting on my tits!

④ A breast pump is the closest I'll get to making out with a robot!

ERR ERR ERR

Pumping is tough, though. Whoever said, 'Don't cry over spilt milk' has never accidentally knocked over a bottle of expressed breastmilk. Despite the fact that I wasn't getting a lot of milk out, my boobs were still leaking every time the babies cried, even when they weren't crying because they were hungry.

22 August

When Colm is at work I spend all day with the babies. My wit is wasted on them – their interests are drinking milk and crying as a form of artistic expression – and time with them is intense. Firstly there are two of them and you cannot make small talk with a newborn – they have no concept of the news, the weather or Joe Duffy. They also don't understand that maybe you would like to sleep for more than two hours at a time, or that perhaps they could wait their turn to cry.

When Colm comes home I ask him about the adult world, update him on how much poo has been created, and try to pawn off something I heard on the radio as my own news. I think being busy is good because the times I'm not busy, I'm filled with worries that I'm not doing things right or that something is wrong. For example, when they're sleeping:

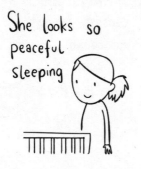

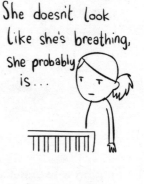

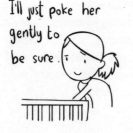

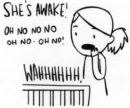

THIS BUT LOTS OF TIMES

24 August

Today we tried 'no-nappy time'. A time for babies to just chill out without the constraints of nappies. I left Colm with the commando squad and started cooking. He finally came downstairs, carrying one twin, and said, 'Right, after you left, the peeing started. They both ended up damp and unhappy. It wasn't a success.'

25 August

Emma from work had her baby – a little girl, too. It feels weird to be slightly ahead of someone else having a baby – she had been stuck feeling massive and crap and still pregnant, and I've been trying to wrangle two newborns, feeling like the massive-and-crap stage maybe wasn't so bad after all. It was bad, though.

I told her I really enjoy being able to lie on my back in bed again, even if it's only for an hour and a half at a time. We now text each other about how bloody weird this all is.

27 August

The twins are six weeks old today.

I was holding Bronagh after the morning feed, and sat her up to wind her. Then I turned her to face Colm, who was holding Róisín. I like to use the babies as staring ventriloquist dummies, putting a finger and thumb on their chubby wee cheeks to make their mouths open and close. Much of the time I do this while performing a Richard Nixon impression.

'I am not a crook! I am a baby! I have not pooped my pants!'

Today I did it and sang some Cutting Crew, Bronagh's wee face lip syncing and facing our audience.

Colm said, 'She's loving that.'

I turn her towards me and do it again. She has a

huge smile on her face.

It doesn't work the third time.

Even amazing comedy has its limits.

Bronagh is suddenly a bit of craic.

She smiles as I play with her. Róisín cries. I tell Colm that I think Róisín might have pooed, and he offers to swap babies so that I can check.

No poo, but now Colm has Bronagh.

Colm has 'Fun Baby'.

Róisín isn't there yet. She spits up and cries.

Colm plays with Bronagh while grinning at me.

'Awwww... Fun Baby.'

I put Róisín in a sling, carry her around the house, and she falls asleep against me.

She'll catch up.

Now I realize the reason that people say 'the first six weeks are the hardest' isn't because the rest of this parenting lark is easy, it's that things become more rewarding.

31 August

Yesterday I admitted I am depressed.

I said the words tearfully to Colm after walking into the room and giving him a look that prompted an 'Are you OK?' from him.

I am not OK.

Before the twins were born I had no real expectations of what motherhood would be like. I certainly did not think the reality would be the incredible time and personality vacuum in which I'm finding myself. I feel lost in it.

I am not myself. My energy and time are given to the thankless care of two infants. When they were born I was assured that the first six weeks would be the hardest. Unbeknown to those people who told me that, their words gave me something to look forward to: the

THE DREADED COLIC

Colic is when a baby cries for more than three hours, three times a week for three weeks, and seemingly for no reason. A description that does nothing to change my husband's thoughts on the matter: 'I don't think anyone actually knows what colic is. I think they just made it up so that when a baby's been crying for hours, you can say, "It must be colic!"'

He said it in frustration because the babies had been crying for four hours. When they cried so loud and for so long, I wanted to help them but I couldn't. I also wanted to get away from the din but I couldn't because I would be holding one of them. Sometimes I would be holding both, which meant I got the noise in stereo. It felt like being in a house when the intruder alarm goes off, but it's your own house and no one knows the code to silence it.

That space – when you're holding a crying baby who wants you to make them feel better, but you feel powerless because you can't, and all you can do is try to soothe them as they emit their incredibly loud noise to tell you they aren't OK – is difficult to exist in, and at the same time feels like your entire existence.

The colic remedies and potions didn't help and compounded my husband's belief that it is a made-up word simply to give a name to the incredible force of a baby crying for hours on end. To reassure you that you aren't going mad when all evidence points to the fact that the baby has been crying for so long that maybe you are.

In actual fact, research has indicated that colic is the result of a newborn's gut becoming populated by bacteria which is moving in and getting excited about its new home. And we all know it takes some time for a new neighbourhood to settle. All of which is lost on a colicky baby who just wants to be held, and its parents who just want the noise to stop. And eventually it does.

six-week mark. The babies are now almost seven weeks old and it feels as if there is only more of the same ahead.

My days without Colm are spent mostly in the twins' bedroom, as it's easiest to deal with them there. Between the times I'm with them, I clean bottles or dishes or clothes, try to clean the house, make up bottles, and try to feed myself. Right now they have just woken, are gurgling, and I feel the tension in my neck increasing as I'm waiting for one of them to start crying.

Some days Colm has come home and asked me how I am and I've cried. Other days I've warned him that I'm going to leave the room as soon as he comes home. Other days are fine. They bleed into one another because of the night feeds and being awake on and off when I should be asleep. Days do not feel like they truly end.

In the past six and a bit weeks, I have been out by myself – without the twins, for any length of time – just four times. One of those times I registered their birth and had coffee with a friend. I called Colm while I was out and he was trying to deal with them both while working.

I find this is the hard part. I know I should step away but it's hard to hand them off to someone at a time when you know they're at their busiest. It's like handing someone a bomb after the fuse has already been lit.

Colm doesn't mind, but I find myself thinking, 'I'm finding this so hard and this is all I have to do!' It feels wrong to burden him with this level of solo parenting on top of the responsibility he has with his job. As their mum, I feel as if I should be the person doing it all. It's what I signed up for, after all. And there are also hormones – so many hormones – telling me that I have to stay and be near the babies at all times.

So the last few weeks have been a slow burn of cabin fever. Babies are not easy company and aren't relaxing to be around. Have you ever been in a situation where you're talking to someone and feel you've to carry the entire conversation? That's babies. Silent, staring. Then their face crinkles – they're going to cry. Don't cry. You jiggle them. Don't cry. The other one cries – the one you're not holding. Jesus Christ.

Before I was a mother, I was someone else. I was a scientist, but then these guys were born and my work haven't even sent me a card. I've worked there seven years. I'm on maternity leave, I haven't ceased to exist. It makes me feel that now I'm a mother, I'm not a scientist. I'm not me. I don't know who I am.

All of this – spiralling feelings of being trapped, self-doubt and anxiety – is further fuelled by lack of sleep. There are moments where I think, 'I could have a nap' but I find myself just lying there, tense, staring at the ceiling, waiting for one of the babies to cry.

In fact, one of them just woke up, so she is now perched awkwardly on me as I try to finish writing this.

I am making arrangements to talk to someone. I have to do something. I can't go on feeling like this. I want to be a good mother and wife and friend, but I need to sort myself out first.

This isn't who I am.

I'm just a bit lost.

POSTPARTUM CHANGES AKA META-MOM-PHOSIS

I didn't know who I was any more. Becoming a mother had changed me in a number of ways. First, there were the physical changes...

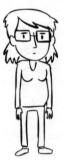

WHAT MY BODY LOOKED LIKE AFTER GIVING BIRTH.

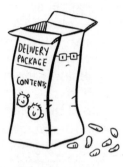

WHAT IT FELT LIKE

My body felt like a package that had contained a delivery of babies, or a rented house after the tenants had moved out. It didn't feel like mine any more and was a bit wrecked. I'd predicted that you can't blow up a balloon and expect it not to be changed by the experience a bit when it eventually deflates. What I hadn't predicted was how those changes would make me feel. I thought that having the babies would be like when we got the cat. They would be something we would look after, and although we would probably be really tired we could at least stop dressing the cat like a baby (kidding).

continued...

I realized something was up. Their cries wrenched me physically, my new drinks-dispenser boobs were holding happy hour in response, and if I was asleep and the babies woke up I'd know they were awake before they even cried. I thought that was pretty normal. Then Colm went out to meet his friends and came back.

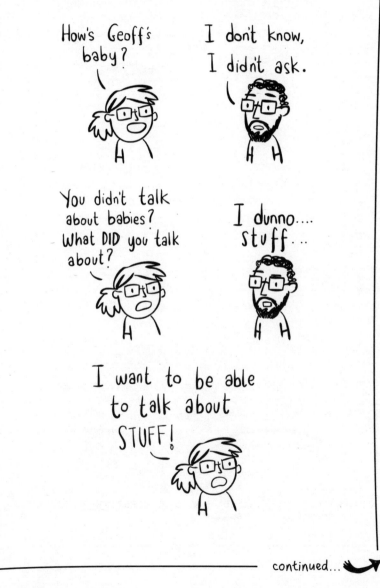

continued...

That's because my social interactions were:

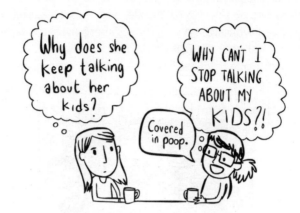

When people say 'parenthood has changed me', they aren't being glib. It actually changes you. Your body doesn't trust you to look after babies, having only skimmed a parenting book and owned a cat that the vet thinks has exceptionally clean teeth, so it alters how you think by physically changing your brain. I'm realizing now that this sounds really ominous, but my brain wanted me to be weirdly obsessed with my kids. However, although I was weirdly obsessed with my kids, I didn't know what was happening to who I used to be or if she'd ever come back.

Before I became a parent my mind was a mixture of

work FOOD SCIENCE L♥VE TV MOVIES HOME FRIENDS ART

BUT AFTERWARDS IT WAS LIKE

BABIES L♥VE FOOD WASHING CLOTHES "Can I die from being this tired?!"

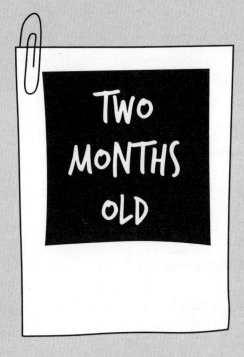

16 SEPTEMBER - 15 OCTOBER

* Coos, gurgles and makes other
  vocal sounds

* Sees black-and-white patterns

* Follows objects across field of vision

* Discovers hands

* Holds head up for short periods of time

* Smiles and laughs

* Briefly grasps and holds objects
  placed in hand

18 September

My mum told me she got a new washing machine.
I asked how long she had had the old one.

'Fourteen years.'

'Wow. That's a long time.'

'I know. I was wondering if I'd be alive long enough to need another one.'

'That's great. You're thinking of your life in terms of the washing machine and not whether or not you'll see your grandkids grow up.'

'But I see the washing machine every day!'

19 September

I talked to my counsellor today. She describes herself as a counsellor but I call her 'the lady I cry in front of who isn't allowed to feel awkward about it'. I first started seeing her three years ago. It wasn't because of one particular thing – or because things got bad – but because things could be better. I thought that she would take years of accumulated emotional baggage and make it all go away but what actually happened was that she helped me to slowly unpack everything I was carrying. Then we figured out how much I needed to keep with me and how it could feel lighter or be carried more effectively. It didn't stop me talking to other people about my problems either, it just helped me to express them better.

The last time I saw her was during the pregnancy and we tried to untangle my feelings about it. I now see her only when things are bad, and they aren't great at the moment. We talk about what is happening and how I am tired – it's difficult to articulate properly. She says I should come back and I say I will. However, it's hard; it's hard for me to step away like this and take some time for myself, which is probably part of the problem.

20 September

During the week, when I'm flying solo with the babies, my life exists within a 'zone of parenting confidence'. It's an area where I am happy to bring them, safe in the knowledge that I can also get home quickly. I am living my life between feeds: I feed them, try to get them into the buggy and get out before coming back for the next feed.

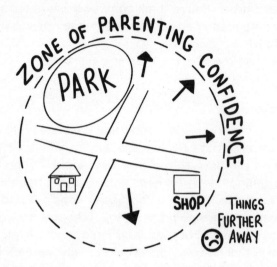

The downside about the park is that other mothers could be there with their new babies. Those mums look more together, with their sunglasses and brushed hair, and outfits that aren't just a hoodie and non-maternity jeans. They look like yummy mummies while I look like an au pair that hasn't passed a background check.

I have no idea what to wear as my body hasn't gone back to what it used to look like, so a large number of items in my wardrobe don't fit me. I've basically been dressing like a hobo for this past while. Any time I go shopping I buy baby clothes in the hope that people will see only the babies and not me. Babies are masters of distraction, you see. Magicians' assistants for people who want to disappear socially.

I've discovered that older ladies in particular love babies. A double buggy is like a Kinder Surprise to them – they can't wait to see what's inside. In the beginning I found this strange, but the conversations have become predictable – not in the sense that I could tell when they would happen, but that people have similar questions each time.

Some of these silver-haired ladies have got to know me and I've got to know them, and sometimes we say

Conversations with Strangers when you have twins in a buggy BINGO!!!

"Are they twins?"	Tries to guess their sex	GETS IT WRONG	"How old are they?"	You can't remember how old they are.
"What are their names?"	"Those are lovely names."	Asks you to repeat one of the names	You repeat both names	"Are they identical?"
"Are they identical?" after you've said they're a girl + boy	"How do you tell them apart?"		"Double trouble!"	"Two for the price of one."
"How are they sleeping?"	"You must be exhausted?"	"Do twins run in the family?"	You try to explain the science of twins.	You just say "yes" because it's easier.
They try to make the babies smile.	One baby cries.	Both babies cry.	Compliment on your parenting skillz!	"Enjoy them, they grow up so fast"

95

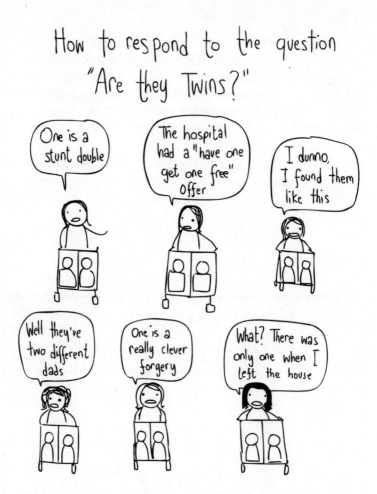

How to respond to the question "Are they Twins?"

hello to each other or smile. I'm no longer invisible in the big city. I'm no longer the person keeping mostly to herself, wearing headphones on the bus and just existing in a house in the area where she lives. I've somehow become part of the community – like a character in a story – except I don't have my own name, I have an occupation, which is 'the lady with the twins'.

I've started to measure my days by how many adult conversations I have. Small chats with people in the neighbourhood who I don't really know but know enough to say hello. Suddenly Dublin isn't this huge anonymous city, it's a huge anonymous city that contains an area in which I am not anonymous.

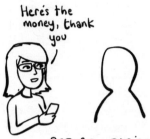

Talking to the person at the checkout.

Here's the money, thank you

BEFORE BABIES

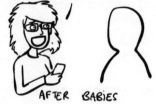

HELLO FELLOW ADULT LET US DISCUSS THINGS THAT ARE UNRELATED TO PARENTING!*

AFTER BABIES

* IT'S A LIE, I'd end up talking about my babies.

22 September

Colm's parents are moving to Carlow. This isn't really news. We've known for a while. They've been running their launderette in Dublin together for years and his mum wants to retire. They live in Finglas, an area of the city which some people would consider rough. People from Finglas would say that Colm's parents live in the posh part.

Colm and I both grew up on housing estates, just at opposite ends of the country. His house is older – his mum grew up in it too – and his family lived with his grandparents until they died. Over the years the house has felt like a home to me too. In it I'd perform the rituals of familiarity usually reserved for my own parents' house. Opening the fridge, for example, and staring at its contents – not because I was hungry but because I wanted to see what was in there.

It feels weird that they're moving. We brought the babies to the house so that when they're older we can tell them that they've been in their father's house even if they don't remember. I took a photo of them there, asleep on their granddad and their uncle. Both babies were dressed in Dublin jerseys that my father-in-law had presented to us when the twins were a day old; just to remind me that my children are from Dublin now.

Colm's mother was getting rid of things in a skip, but keeping things that meant a lot to her: Colm's blue first communion jacket, her children's exam results, some of their childhood comics. Moving everything means digging through the past and wondering which parts to keep, a house of memories either packed into boxes or placed in a skip.

For me, it is a house of memories – of Christmases and birthdays, calling to see Colm's parents, living there when I was between places – but I've only been a visitor there for the past eleven years. I asked Colm if he was sad that his parents were leaving it. He told me that in a way he was, but that it was his parents' place now – not his – and they wanted to retire and move on.

25 September

The babies are ten weeks old now. Every so often I try to push the envelope of my independence with them, ticking off a list of things that feel impossible until attempted. The first of those things was 'leaving the house' – the first time we brought them out in the buggy. Then it was 'take them on a bus' and 'take them out on my own'. Each first attempt at one of these small feats was a moment of intense anxiety. I waited for my children to explode into almighty fireballs and for strangers to point at me while chanting, 'Bad mother! Bad mother!' over and over.

Each time we leave the house it gets a bit easier – by 'easier' I probably mean 'more efficient'. Knowing what to pack – nappies, food, clothes in case they piss all over their current outfit. For me, being organized gives me the illusion that I am somehow in control.

I brought them into town today. I had to run a few errands, and that meant bringing them with me. It was either that or deciding maybe it was high time the cat stepped up to her responsibilities.

I'm beginning to realize that some people really like to hold babies.

'Can I pick her up?' they ask.

Today, other people, who aren't related to me, held the babies and cooed at them, and they smiled back because they're beginning to work the room. I'm unsure what to do with myself when other people have them. I feel like a salesperson in a baby showroom.

'Yes, this is our 2015 model. It's one of a matching pair.'

I also worry that if the baby cries, I'll have to take it back and say, 'Sorry, this one is broken. Let me fetch you another.'

They don't cry, though. Partially because maybe they're having a great day and the people holding them are good with babies, but also because they have soothers.

I could kiss whoever invented soothers, or, as we call them, 'peacekeepers'.

Colm said that there should be something you can use to keep a soother in a baby's mouth at all times. I told him he had basically described a ball-gag.

With all this interaction with other people, I'm beginning to appreciate that some people find genuine joy in babies. Some people don't like them. I see the fear in those people's eyes that I will hand them a baby, or the babies will cry. Much like I used to be. Despite this, I am finding it easier to say 'sure' when someone I know asks to hold them, and also to ask someone to hold them while I try to do something.

And it's fine. The babies don't explode and I don't run away to Cuba.

Still, I haven't taken the twins out and fed them both on my own. Today, my friend Shaun helped. I fed one, he fed the other, then we swapped as his baby started to malfunction and wouldn't take their bottle. By helping me, Shaun allowed his lunch to go cold, before offering me half of it. Small acts such as this make me appreciate people hugely. For them it's a small favour, for me it's an edge off my anxiety. All the while, the infant overlords lazed around, full of milk, and gave gummy smiles to those around them.

Hopefully, one of these days I will manage all this by myself, but right now, being able to ask for and get help feels like something to tick off the list.

27 September

When I hand the babies over to be held, sometimes people say, 'Oh, that new-baby smell!' As if the baby is a car. I'm confused, so I smell their heads.

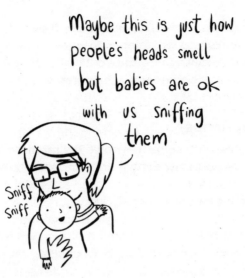

29 September

'Let's get some shots!' I said yesterday in my GP's surgery as the girls got their first vaccinations.

These were the first in a series of immunizations I like to call the 'parenting bonus round'. The needle was so big that if it was scaled up to be used on an adult, it would be a two-person job. I'm all for big pricks but this was ridiculous. I felt bad because my GP is a wonderful woman and she's just made a terrible first impression on my kids. Their reaction to the shot was 'What the feck was that?' as they cried, then sucked anxiously on their soothers before falling asleep.

Later came the 'What the feck is this?' as the vaccination piqued the interest of their immune system and their temperature went up. This called for me to administer Calpol, which was spat out before I realized I could use a soother to trap it in there. Other parents have described infant paracetamol syrup as both 'delicious' and something magical. Inconsolable wailing does not say 'delicious', unless you take that rhyme about screaming for ice cream literally.

They slept eventually and today they definitely seem way less likely to get tetanus from all those rusty nails I've been throwing into their cots.

Good job, babies and attenuated viruses!

30 September

Being a parent seems to involve taking pride in your kid's achievements. Even if one of those achievements is simply 'taking a dump'.

Babies set the bar really low.

I'm waiting for Róisín to poop. She's constipated – again. She isn't happy about it either. Sometimes I wish the solution were simply to give her the magazine section of the weekend *Guardian* and twenty minutes' privacy.

This has made me realize something. No matter what you have or haven't achieved in your life, try to remember that at some point someone in your life was incredibly proud of you for taking a dump.

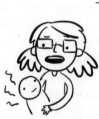

BABY POOS DEFY PHYSICS!

THIS BABY HAS POOED UP ITSELF! THAT'S RIGHT – UP!

2 October

After the 5.30 a.m. feed this morning, the babies were awake. Róisín has started making this cat-like howling noise to let us know that she is awake and bored.

Bored?!

It's 5.30 a.m. Nothing is happening.

5.30 a.m. is boring. That's why there's this thing called sleep.

Both babies ended up in the bed with us. Before today, if we brought them into the bed, they would fall asleep and we would fall asleep, holding their delicate bodies protectively. It was pretty sweet.

This morning, however, Bronagh's flailing hands smacked me in the face at irregular intervals. Róisín squirmed on Colm's chest and made grunting noises. This did not stop.

There was no sleep.

Colm got up for work, put Róisín back in the cot and she grinned a big, gummy grin at him.

'"Let's have babies," you said. "It'll be fun," you said,' I mumbled as Bronagh backhanded my nose for the fiftieth time.

3 October

Bronagh just flipped from her front to her back. She's eleven weeks old. I think this is an achievement for her because it took a number of attempts and when she finally managed it she burst into tears.

It was a bit like Rocky Balboa crying out, 'ADRIAAAAAAN!' after he won his fight at the end of the movie.

Except way, way, way less exciting. Unless you're Colm or myself.

Róisín puked up milk on me and her socks. Right now the movie she's channelling is *The Exorcist*.

4 October

We are each holding a baby.

'Colm, which baby is your favourite today?'

'This one.'

'Because you're holding her?'

'Because I'm holding her, because she finished her bottle and because your one kicked me in the balls earlier.'

Parenting: the good days are good. The bad days remind you how tough it gets and you feel like an idiot for thinking the good days will last.

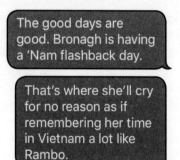

The good days are good. Bronagh is having a 'Nam flashback day.

That's where she'll cry for no reason as if remembering her time in Vietnam a lot like Rambo.

5 October

Yesterday, Bronagh had one of her ''Nam flashback' days. Today, it's Róisín's turn.

It's 10 a.m. and I am knackered.

I suggested that we all have a lazy day. Róisín's response involved crying as she suddenly recalled a chopper exploding and burning metal raining into the thick jungle canopy.

7 October

Right now I'm the babies' favourite person. I've an adoring fan club of two.

Benedict Cumberbatch could walk into this room but all eyes would be on me.

The babies' eyes because I'm their favourite, and Benedict Cumberbatch's because I'd imagine he'd feel incredibly confused.

Then I'd make him help me feed them.

9 October

I bought a ticket for the Euromillions draw tonight. I don't play it that often, but each time I fully expect to win it. To such a degree that I don't look forward to the draw, I look forward to collecting the money. When I don't win, the loss is so crushing that I don't play it for at least another six months.

I'm not paying for a ticket, you see. I'm paying for a few days of fantasy, and the only cheque I get to cash is a reality cheque.

So, Colm is losing his job.

A couple of years ago, Colm worked for a company which then closed its Dublin office. It was really stressful. He lost his job, then our landlady decided to sell the house we were renting, so we had to move. After not being able to find a place for some time, we eventually did.

I was really f**king stressed. It was hard.

Colm took a job at a company he didn't like. He hated the job and he hated the company. When they downsized their offices, he was happy to leave. He started working part time for another company and enjoyed it. It was meant to become a full-time position but that's not happening now. It's more likely to become 'no time'.

The stress I feel about this, I found out today, is fluctuating. Plus point: Colm gets to see more of the babies growing up. Minus point: no job.

I also didn't win the Euromillions. C'mon, Fate, gimme a break!

10 October

This morning I was dressing the babies as Colm went downstairs to iron his shirt. I was singing them a song – which I do a lot, like a slightly manic Mary Poppins. This one was about dresses and tights.

Colm was taking his sweet time and we had to leave,

so I went to the bedroom door and called out, 'COLM? What's taking so long?'

'Sorry, I'm ironing, washing, getting dressed and stuff...' he called back.

Then there was a pause.

'...I think the cat may have cornered a mouse in the dining room.'

The babies were placed unceremoniously back in their cots and I rushed downstairs.

'Where is it?'

'Under the bookcase. The cat was pawing under it and I heard squeaking.'

I got down on my stomach, Colm handed me a bike light and I peered under the furniture.

'Colm, that's not a mouse. It's a rat.'

A sudden rush of urgency was injected into the situation.

'Get the hoover!' I demanded.

'You're going to suck it out?'

'That, or scare it out! Then the cat can get it!'

As soon as Colm brought the vacuum cleaner into the room the cat started to panic.

'Oh, f**k. I forgot – she hates it! Get it out! Get it out!'

The cat was now no longer interested in the rat and simply wanted to leave. We looked around the room for something to poke the rat out with. There was nothing. We needed a broom; we also needed the cat. I held her, reassuring her that she could do this, while Colm got the floor brush.

Now armed with the brush, I confronted the rat. I poked it with the broom handle and it squeaked and moved out of its hiding place between the bookcase and the corner of the wall to further under the bookcase. Dragging the handle across the floor I crowded the squeaking rat out from under its literary lair. When its body was mostly exposed we fetched the cat.

We put her beside the rat, which was trying to conceal itself by hiding its head.

And. She. Did. Nothing.

'F**k my life,' I said, asking Colm for the hand towel beside him.

'F**k my life,' I repeated, picking up the squirming rat in the towel.

'F**k my life!'

Carrying it through the kitchen and out the back door.

'F**k my life!'

Following Colm, I walked across the wet grass in my socks to throw the rat out the back gate, which Colm held open.

Looking confused as it landed, it got up and scurried away.

'This is too much for a Saturday morning.'

And I then asked Colm if I was his hero. He told me that he would have picked up the rat too. Actually, his idea had been to trap it under a bowl, as if it were a spider, but I didn't say that.

'Just say, "You're my hero!"'

'You're my hero.'

'I know.'

14 October

In the last two months I have taken an insane number of photos of these children and maybe three photos of myself. I have also taken a number of pictures of Colm and our children – mostly in the classic dad-is-asleep-and-babies-are-asleep pose – which are super cute but they also mean *I'm* not asleep.

WHY I TAKE MORE PHOTOS OF MY KIDS THAN MYSELF

 Their clothes look cute and fit them

 Mine don't

They're happy and well rested

Can I die from being this tired?

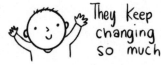 They keep changing so much.

 I've worn the same hoodie for a week!

I love them and want to hold on to the moments that I can't actively enjoy.

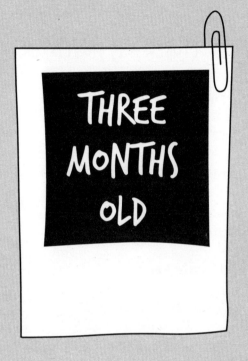

16 OCTOBER – 15 NOVEMBER

* Smiles and laughs

* Holds head steady

* Imitates some movements and
    facial expressions

* Brings hand to mouth

* Blows bubbles

* Knows parent's face

* Lifts head and shoulders when lying
    on tummy

* Supports upper body with arms
    when lying on tummy

18 October

So yesterday I thought I might have Colm's cold. I was so wrong.

I got it today. So did my brood. They aren't dealing with it very well.

It must be tough – they're trying to get to grips with their bodies and have only just stopped smacking themselves in the face with their own hands. Now they've a cold. Something new, something unpleasant, and it's ruined their not-smacking-myself-in-my-face-with-my-own-hand streak.

I've discovered that 'What the f**k is happening to me?' in baby-speak equates to constant crying. Baby seems to be a tonal language, something I'm appreciating now as they rest against my chest, head beside my ear, bellowing their displeasure like the Linguaphone CD from hell.

I have filled them full of Calpol, which although it does not contain sugar, is somehow so sticky that when they bat themselves in the face repeatedly it sounds like someone filling in a Panini World Cup 2014 sticker album.

I have told them, 'I also have a cold, but you don't see me crying.'

That's because I eat my feelings.

19 October

The public health nurse called to check the babies and to patronize me with advice on how not to kill them. We found out that Bronagh is bigger and stronger than Róisín, a fact that was discovered using weighing scales and by placing them on their stomachs.

It should have been decided in battle: the best of three rounds.

The victor gets to beat up a car.

The nurse said that we need to make Róisín stronger.

I'm going to help Róisín to do this in a montage set to an eighties power ballad. Meanwhile, Bronagh will be observed by people with clipboards on a playmat in a state-of-the-art gym in Soviet Russia.

ADULT TRAINING MONTAGE

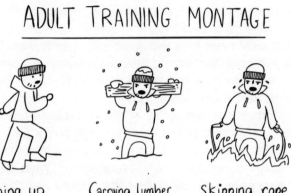

Running up lots of steps

Carrying lumber in the snow

Skipping rope in a fire

BABY TRAINING MONTAGE

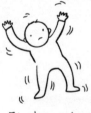

Flailing about

Trying to crush your finger.

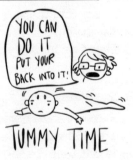

YOU CAN DO IT PUT YOUR BACK INTO IT!

TUMMY TIME

20 October

Today was difficult.

I still have a cold, something which is making me tired. I've had one before, though, so I know what to expect. The babies also still have their colds – their first ever colds – which means their mood switches from fine, to devastated, back to fine again in swift rotation.

They cry, are confused by what is happening, tired, irritated and unable to settle. They're unhappy and unwilling to eat, then suddenly hungry and demanding.

Incredibly demanding.

At their best, they are amazing. I didn't anticipate being able to bear witness to how far people come through their lifetime. Observing the twins' intellect blossoming like a flower, their fumbling attempts to master the workings of a body that didn't exist a year ago. The thought that 'I was once like this' bubbles up over and over again.

Demanding babies are hard and, despite myself, I've once again let the amount of time I'm spending with them pile on to me until things have become unbearably difficult.

Colm came home while I was feeding Bronagh and I started to cry.

Róisín, who was beside her sister, looked at me, trying to figure out my facial expression.

'Don't f**k up your kids! Don't f**k up your kids!' a voice in my head shouted, causing me to force a smile and sing to her.

'I need to get away for a bit,' I said to Colm as he rubbed my shoulders. 'A few hours. Just away from this. I've been in the house for two days. I've not gone anywhere on my own, that wasn't for some practical reason, in three weeks.'

'I know. Go to the cinema. We need to make time for this. Once a week.'

We say this, but we are bad at making it happen.

It will get better. I'm finding that I have to step away, and things won't implode when I do. Colm is able to handle his brood.

So today I paid for a taxi to the cinema, a ticket, some

ice cream, a drink, a taxi home, and I bought Colm and
I burritos on the way back because we needed to eat.

The bottom line is, I paid a lot of money to be on my
own for four hours.

And it was totally worth it.

25 October

The babies love to projectile vomit on to Colm.

On this occasion it was like a gunge tank from an
eighties game show, right against his chest.

Baby vomit is the least offensive kind of vomit. It
goes baby vomit, cat vomit, then adult vomit. You clean
up the first two without much grumbling, but the third
one stinks and you do feel that maybe you shouldn't
even be helping because the culprit is neither a baby
nor a cat.

Incidentally, dogs clean up their own vomit. As if
their stomach spilled its contents inadvertently the same
way you might drop change out of a purse accidentally.

'Oops! My bad! I'll just get that.'

26 October

Ever since they were born, the babies have pretty much
ignored the hell out of each other, like two women
wearing the same dress at a party. However, political
relations between the babies have begun to thaw
recently. It started with one staring intensely at the
other while she was looking away, otherwise known as
the ABBA effect.

Last night, after one of the feeds, Colm and I held
them in bed, sitting them on the edge of our stomachs.
We've propped them up in this way before, to no avail.
They stared at us, the lamp, the wall, back at us, gave a
quick glance at the other baby, then stared back at us
again.

HOW YOU EXPECT TWIN BABIES TO INTERACT

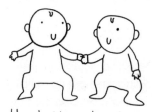

Sweetly holding hands gazing
at each other, smiling, best friends

HOW THEY ACTUALLY INTERACT

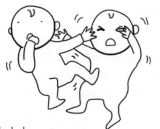

Completely ignoring each other as
they flail around until one accidentally
smacks the other in the face. Both cry

Today something has changed, though. I held Róisín and Colm was holding Bronagh. They stared – just like before – except this time at each other. Unblinking, intense eye contact.

Colm and I could see only the face of the baby the other was holding.

'Róisín is smiling at Bronagh,' Colm said.

'Well, Bronagh is smiling right back.'
Brief, warm smiles at 'the other baby'.
It felt like the end of the divide and the start of 'them'.
Though it might just have been wind.

28 October

Since the babies have started to acknowledge the other's existence, we've been playing 'the other baby' regularly.

This involves each of us holding one twin and making them face each other while saying, 'Look at the other baby!'

There has been an exchange of smiles but today there was an exchange of gurgles. Colm said, 'Look, they're starting their secret language.'

Which made it creepy.

30 October

Of all the weird side effects I had while I was pregnant, I actually liked the fact that my hair stopped falling out.

No red hairs on hair brushes, the carpet or, most importantly, in the plug hole. Today I noticed that that period of hair hoarding has ended. I picked a lump of sodden hair from the plug hole and threw it into the composting bag in the kitchen.

'You can't compost hair!' Colm said.

'You can! It's hair!'

'No. It doesn't break down. Like those skulls in *Indiana Jones* – they had bits of hair on them.'

'It has to break down. It's organic.'

'But worms break down the compost. You don't want a worm working away, then it gets one of your hairs caught in its mouth and it's, like, "Gak! Gak!" But it can't remove it as it has no hands.'

'Fine, I'll take it out.'

31 October

Babies don't need Hallowe'en outfits, as children are generally quite scary already, and it turns out that Hallowe'en costumes are not a baby's outfit of choice. They don't care that it's their first Hallowe'en or that my mother-in-law bought them outfits. They don't care that they look super cute.

The photo below is meant to give the impression that they're going to be wee pumpkins all day.

In reality, how long were they dressed like this? Ten minutes.

I knew as soon as I dressed Bronagh in her outfit that she hated it. Róisín was a bit happier – it was her time to shine, wearing something as big and as orange as the sun. While I'm setting them down against their emergency-foil-poncho background, my husband is asking what I want for breakfast and I'm shouting, 'I don't care. I need to take this photo before all hell breaks loose!'

I take a few snaps.

Sure, this isn't a photo of two smiling babies but I like it because Róisín is who we all want to be at a Hallowe'en party, but Bronagh is who we actually are.

At three months old, she's already too old for this shit.

Shit that she lost completely as I took the outfit off her.

Happy Hallowe'en.

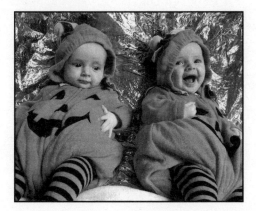

Hallowe'en fireworks are being set off outside.

The noise shakes the single glazing of our windows.

The bangs have resulted in both babies having severe Vietnam flashbacks. One minute they're trying to sleep in their cot, the next their platoon falls under heavy gunfire. Bodies are scattered, dog tags are in the dirt. They pick up the tags, shove them in their mouths and cry loudly.

Back in their cot, they suck their fists in the darkness. Colm and I each comfort a baby. During this time Colm also remakes a cup of tea three times. It goes cold each time, the heat seeping from it, as from the bodies of the lost on the Ho Chi Minh trail.

HOW TO TAKE A GREAT BABY PHOTO

① Take a photo.

② Look at it.

③ Move all the junk out of shot to give the illusion that your house isn't complete chaos.

④ Retake photo.

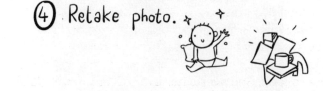

2 November

Róisín has been cooing for a few weeks now, which involves her making a very soft 'oooo' noise. She coos when I sing to her. She coos at her bear. When she wants attention and she's in the cot, though, she yells. You go and look at her and she starts cooing again while smiling. She has a delicate and girly voice – almost musical.

For a few weeks Bronagh has been relatively silent. She has cried when upset and smiled when happy. I was worried, worried that she was going to be the quiet one. Not speaking, just smiling and nodding.

Today Bronagh found her voice.

It is not an inside one.

It is not delicate or girly. It is Bronagh's voice.

She yells.

She yells at her bear. She yells when she wants attention. You go and look at her and she yells at you while smiling.

It's like living with a football fan!

'Mum, we do. Mum, we do. Mum, we do. Oh, Mum, we love you!'

4 November

Bronagh is continuing in her endeavour to communicate. She's decided that volume is key; the louder the better. Her favourite noise to make is an 'OOOH OOOH WOOOH', which makes her sound less like a monkey and more like someone trying to offend a monkey. She makes this noise at us, at toys and at Róisín.

Now, when Bronagh first looks at Róisín, Róisín smiles, then Bronagh smiles. Then, Bronagh starts with the 'OOOH OOOH WOOOH' and Róisín doesn't know where to look. She averts her eyes as you might do if an elderly relation made an outburst containing the phrase 'Feck off back to where they came from!'

Bronagh continues to stare at Róisín, making her noise with a look that suggests, 'C'mon, you know this one! Sing along!' Like an entertainer on a cruise ship.

I'm hoping that 'OOOH OOOH WOOOH' doesn't catch on.

6 November

In Tesco, the amount of cat hair on my coat suggests to other shoppers that I am single. However, the baby formula I'm buying suggests that either I have a baby or things are getting weird with the cat.

10 November

I decided to give Bronagh some baby rice this morning. Baby rice is basically a way of thickening milk, and this prepares babies for the wonder of actual food.

Firstly, Bronagh did not want the baby rice as food. She wanted to hold it in her mouth before pushing it out of her milk-hole with her tongue. Then she shoved her fist into her mouth, covered it in baby rice and wiped it everywhere, before she tried to push all of her bib into her face.

The whole thing felt like the miracle of the loaves and the fishes: the two spoonfuls I gave her seemed to multiply in her mouth. Unless she's actually a bottomless baby-rice dispenser.

Afterwards, I had to clean her and make her a bottle to both wash the rice out of her mouth and bribe her for her love.

In conclusion: baby rice can f**k off for a few weeks.

11 November

When Colm's parents were having a clear-out before they moved house, Colm's dad gave me a plasma ball from the contents cull. I plugged it in, placed my hands on the glass, and as its glowing tendrils reached out to meet my skin, I marvelled at it. Colm explained how it worked and I said, 'The babies will love this!'

Today I showed it to Bronagh.

She looked at it

Then tried to eat it

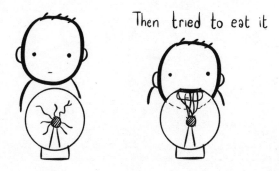

I thought she would find it amazing, but then realized that there are so many new things for them in the world, everything must be amazing right now, and one of the best things about being a parent is becoming their tour guide to it all.

The world has become new again because I'm being forced to look at all of the minute details that make it up; things that I'm so used to seeing that I no longer engage with them. I pick up daisies and blades of grass, point out clouds and drops of rain, and help the babies get to grips with all the small things because they can't see the bigger picture.

It strikes me that our understanding of the world is an accumulation of concepts, each built on top of the others. I went to the cinema to see *Mad Max: Fury Road*, and the idea of even beginning to explain that to a baby becomes huge. It's a movie set in the future, in a desert and people drive large trucks. How do I explain what the

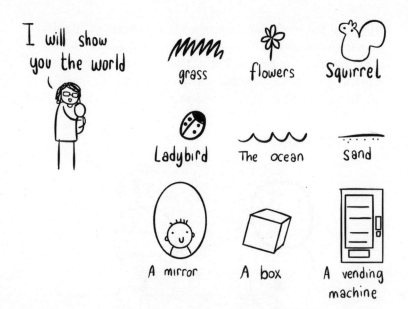

future is? Or a desert? They haven't even seen sand. Also, they won't be able to watch that movie for nearly another eighteen years.

I realize that I don't have to show my kids the entire world. I can start with the park at the end of the road, and not the entire park, just a tree, and not even the whole tree, just a leaf, and we'll work our way up from there.

After I've stopped them trying to eat it.

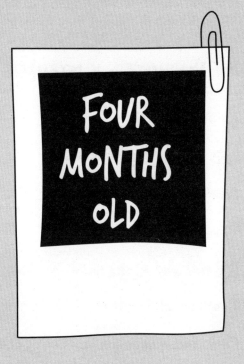

FOUR
MONTHS
OLD

16 NOVEMBER – 15 DECEMBER

* Begins reaching

* Uses arms simultaneously

* Grasps and releases toys

* Brings hands together

* Relaxes and opens hands at rest

* Bears weight on legs

* Coos and makes noise when spoken to

* Rolls over from tummy to back

16 November

Yesterday a friend of mine had a baby shower for her bump. It's a boy. There were Post-it notes for us to write down pieces of parenting advice. Luckily, she found my advice funny.

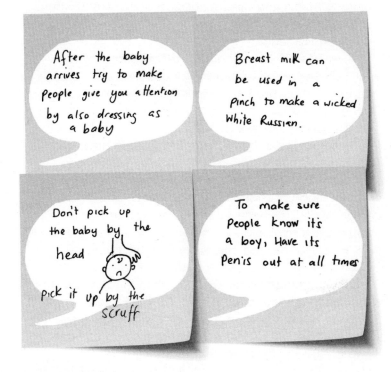

18 November

When I'm walking the babies in the buggy, it's as if I'm in my own version of the movie *Speed*.

If the buggy stops, the babies cry.

If the buggy slows down, the babies cry.

And that bit when Keanu spits out his soother accidentally, doesn't have the requisite limb control to retrieve it and bursts into tears. Then when Sandra Bullock tries to put it back and he keeps sucking her hand instead.

19 November

Colm is away for three days with a bit of work, to fill in the gap of having no work. My parents visit for the day – just for a few hours as they have to go back up to Donegal. My father is only in the door five minutes, holding Róisín and talking absolute shite to her, when she laughs.

A proper laugh.

She has never laughed like that before.

I cry because it is wonderful and new and because I am incredibly tired and tiredness makes me overfeel my emotions.

Do I feel threatened? Yes.

I want my children to laugh at me and now I feel as if they're humouring me. It's like my stuff is good for a gummy smile and a bit of a squeal but, you know, it's not laugh-out-loud funny for them. Also, it's hard to bring your A-game when you're tired as f**k from looking after twins on your own.

Honestly, though, this is my own fault. I haven't been upping my game, my material is stale and they *are* just humouring me. They like the old favourites but they also want something new. They want whatever it is my dad has going on, my dad on the brink of a sell-out nursery tour. My dad who only months ago had cancer and is enjoying his new lease of life.

My dad only has one arm, which sounds like the start of a joke to which the punchline could be 'he's 'armless' but it's not. He lost the other one in an accident on a fishing trawler when he was eighteen and afterwards he went to a stay in lodgings while being rehabilitated. It was there that he met my mum, who was staying there too because she had severe asthma. He took her breath away, which wasn't difficult at the time.

The fact is, if my dad hadn't lost his arm, he wouldn't have met my mum and I wouldn't exist and neither would my kids. Until I was three I believed that all dads had only one arm because he was just like every other dad I knew, doing things such as going to work and telling bad jokes. It's never really held him back but it's difficult to manage babies when you've only one arm, especially when there are two of them. So he doesn't feed the twins, or change them, or wind them. (He mostly says to my mum, 'I think this baby needs to be fed,' then suggests a bit of an egg.) But my god, he's got skills in entertaining them.

I phone Colm and tell him about Róisín laughing. He's happy but disappointed he missed it. I tell him that Bronagh didn't laugh as much or in the same way, so we still have a chance with her. Her laughter cherry is still intact.

That's right, on Saturday we are going to try to make Bronagh laugh properly.

We still have a chance with Fun Baby.

I should have known that Dry Baby would love dad jokes.

Oh, Dry Baby.

20 November

It's now 4.30 a.m. Welcome to early morning 'Nightfeeds'. I am your sole host, Maria, as my regular co-host, Colm, is currently enjoying a full night's sleep in a hotel. GOOD FOR HIM.

In this edition: pooing mid-nappy change. Will this get Bronagh thrown out of the Magic Circle? And Róisín, has she pooed today? I can't remember. Will I worry about that later? Probably.

This, and more, with our resident house band Two Baby Mobiles Playing Different Songs at the Same Time. Welcome to 'Nightfeeds'.

21 November

Some days I feel like a Las Vegas cabaret act when I'm entertaining the babies. It's daytime – I refuse to work at night, and the late-night crowd are the worst. Doing my shtick, I go through the motions, mostly singing, or telling fart jokes.

I wonder if I'm better than this.

Sometimes the entire audience falls asleep.

When this happens I leave the stage and go and get a drink.

Other times, all the audience wants to do is drink, and they get rowdy until that happens.

They piss themselves regularly. This is no reflection on the quality of my act.

They also roll about on the floor. This is not accompanied by laughter.

The only upside is, I am their favourite comic and singer right now. They don't know anyone better and they keep coming back, day after day.

One day I'll take it on tour.

22 November

For weeks, if you were to put your hand near the babies' mouths, it was always the same.

'Awwww, look, she's trying to suck my finger. That's so cute. She thinks I've finger nipples.'

But now it's different.

'Awwww...Wait, she's trying to bite me! That baby is a maniac!'

When they're around four months old, babies become like zombies determined to chew those close to them, as if that will somehow turn their victim into one of them. They may even gum you for hours, trying in vain to break your skin and getting increasingly frustrated in the process.

The infectious-baby phase lasts for a number of

months during which time the baby runs an intermittent fever, has red cheeks and tries to sink its budding gnashers into anything it can get its hands on.

Eventually, it understands that human flesh won't sate its urges, only rusks and other baby mush, and they come to realize that being a teething baby is a bit crap.

25 November

I took the babies for a walk in the park today. It was morning, they were grumbling and I just wanted a bit of peace, so off we went. There are small seagulls in the park – not the big massive bastards from the tabloids, the ones who steal packets of crisps from shops, just small ones. I like to feed them as I'm walking with the buggy, casually dropping food as I go so that it looks as if they're following me. As if we're in my own version of *The Birds*.

Colm had been practising driving with his uncle and they met us in the park. I kept making the birds crowd around us so we were all drawn into my Hitchcockian fantasy and afterwards we went home.

When we arrived I noticed straight away that there was something different about the house.

The front door was wide open.

Wide. Bloody. Open.

I swore in panic and went in to check if anything had been taken.

Nothing, but my heart was pumping. Colm had left the door open by accident.

I was relieved and annoyed and angry, then Colm told me I'd received a letter in the post . . .

My work had written to me to ask if I was coming back after my maternity leave.

I started to cry. Colm asked if it was because he'd left the door open. I said no, it was because of the letter.

I had cried about my work yesterday too, before

the letter came, increasingly aware that I would have to decide what to do before long, about when I should go back.

Colm is still without a job. I've told him we need money and if he doesn't get a job soon, then I'll have to go back early. He thinks he might be getting a job, and if that happens I'll stay home for a few more months. A depressing prospect, to work all day, not to see them and their small progressions, to feel I am missing out.

But babies are boring.

I've been working or studying full time since I was eighteen. I was only without work for one month when I was twenty – the rest is accounted for. I have a degree in science and a PhD, I still work in research as an applied scientist, troubleshooting ideas and working out experiments. It's challenging, but there's no career progression in my current role.

Colm, on the other hand, has gone up and up in his work. Each new job is a new position with more money, more challenges and more development. He is more desirable, more employable.

This is hard. My confidence is shot – both my self-belief and pride in my appearance. Belief and pride require energy but I don't have a lot of energy. I don't have a lot of time to myself to figure out who I am now.

I am aware that this is not a good advert for motherhood.

Having to make the choice between going back to work or being a full-time mother is depressing me. It feels as if I don't have anything to look forward to. People have suggested that I try to make the art work, or write a book, or do both things, or take a course to make myself more employable. Again, all of these things require time and energy, and I don't have a lot of either so now I feel a bit trapped.

Yes, having twins is a bit of an 'instant family', but it's also a great way to take all of your aspirations, put them into a bin, set fire to the bin and then kick it off a cliff.

Even as I write this I can hear Colm trying to stop the babies crying. I'm not going to help. I want him to be aware – painfully aware – of what we are asking me to do, every day, on my own for the next few months.

And I want us to be OK with our decision.

27 November

In the next week Colm will take his driving test. Then, if he doesn't get a job I have to tell my work that I'm going back in the new year.

The babies, who are teething like crazy, are also being baptized next week. It will be the first time our families have come together since our wedding, when my mum was rude to everyone.

Oh, and my brother will be staying with us for three nights, in a house where there's very little room.

And he's bringing his three-year-old son.

I'm sure it will be fine, it just feels like a lot.

29 November

I made Bronagh laugh.

She has never really laughed before and I made her laugh.

I did what all the comedy greats do: they look at life, observe its foibles and distil them into an idea, give a humorous twist to that idea, craft it into a joke, work the joke to make it funnier...

And watch the joke be wasted on a baby who has no real grasp of language. In fact, she can barely grasp a rattle.

So I resorted to bouncing the baby up and down on my stomach while going 'Wooooooo!'

30 November

The babies are getting better at using their feet. Lying on the floor, they push themselves backwards. It reminds me of someone in a horror movie who is running away, falls, then starts trying to escape their doom.

Except the babies end up moving themselves underneath the sofa.

The only solutions to this are:

1. Put socks on their feet to reduce their traction on the playmat. Although they will kick the socks off.

2. Put them in a playpen so that they're contained and every day would be like a WWE cage match. Seriously, I could give each of them an entrance song. I could be one of their managers, Colm could be the other and we could badmouth the rival baby!

3. Remove their feet.

1 December

Colm failed his driving test. It was his first attempt, but he's trying to get his licence to make all of this easier. It feels as if everything is going wrong.

3 December

The last week or so I've cried a lot. Maybe every day. I've cried because I don't feel happy, but sometimes I just feel blank and I want to cry. When I watch TV I hope that an advert will come on that I can cry at, just to have a reason that isn't the all-consuming reason I want to cry.

I think I have pretty bad postnatal depression.

When the twins were seven weeks old I was depressed but that felt like something driven solely by exhaustion and the unrelenting attention that newborns need. I was essentially trapped for weeks on end in one room with crying babies. Then it got better and I thought I had a handle on things; on what I'm meant to do. I'm getting more sleep now – not a lot, but more – and I feel worse.

I've realized in the worst moments that there's nothing in my life to look forward to, just a bleak landscape of more of the same, of my self-confidence shattering into smaller and smaller fragments, of wearing a lot of hoodies.

I love my children.

They are wonderful and amazing.

I know this. I see it in flashes now, not a constant as it used to be. I've been dulled to it. I feel numb.

I'm finding their company difficult and once I cried in front of them. One baby saw me crying and she cried too, unsure what we were crying about but certain it was essential that she also cry. The other noticed that *My Little Pony* was on the TV, which she considers as essential as the news.

I don't feel that I'm meant to go back to work. I feel that I should be the one to raise the twins, but now that it's come down to it, I don't think I can. In my mind, as awful as it would be for them to be raised in a crèche, I think it would be worse for them to be raised by someone who keeps crying in front of them, making them cry too, and becoming blinded to how amazing they are. I don't think the people at the crèche are allowed to cry in front of their charges. They can't – crèches cost so much money the tears would have to be made of diamonds.

This isn't easy. I'm still unsure what to do but I can't continue to feel this low about myself as a wife, as a mother and as a scientist. There is no easy answer. I wish I could just be one of those mothers in picture books, happy making cookies, instead of the one taking a bite out of a cookie as fat tears roll silently down her cheeks and she wonders, 'What the f**k am I doing with my life?'

At the bottom of the page of that particular book, it says F**K and LIFE because kids need to expand their vocabularies.

5 December

In the park, I am walking the buggy and I am crying. I had tried not to but there wasn't anyone around to see me and it's sort of raining so I gave into it and I cried. The babies are sleeping. We are out so they can nap and I'm waiting for Colm. He arrives and I am still crying.

He asks what is wrong, if I'm stressed about the baptism tomorrow.

I do not know what is wrong.

Either I am crying or I am despondent or I am tense.

The other emotions are there but they are muffled. I laugh but I am not joyful, I smile but I am not happy. I thought that deciding to go back to work would put an end to these feelings. It hasn't. I don't know what is wrong.

I want to cry but there is no specific trigger. The need to cry wells up inside me, though. Like a wave it washes over me. I resist it, but after a while it comes back. Sometimes I fight the urge or just give in and cry; other times I cry but feel too tired. It's as if the effort even to make the tears is too much. Apathy against the emotions themselves.

Earlier today I texted my counsellor, asking to talk, to make an appointment. She asked if she could phone me later. I texted back 'yes' and I thanked her. Being around my husband helps – I feel less weighted but then it comes back and I cry and I'm apologizing for crying. I'm asking if I'm a good mother, I'm leaving the room so I'm not crying in front of the children. Worried I'll f**k them up.

The baptism is tomorrow. I do not care. I know

I should be able to enjoy it but the idea of enjoying it seems very distant. Tomorrow I will have to wear a mask of pleasantry over the absolute mess I am right now. I am not looking forward to this. I have nothing suitable to wear. The dresses I wanted to wear do not fit me, because I am not who I was, my body isn't what it was, it is lost. I'll wear the one dress that does fit. Effort.

This all seems like a lot of effort.

I am tired but I have slept.

My counsellor phones me. I cry – no big surprise there. She is silent as I am crying. She asks a question: how am I? In response I cry. I tell her I think I might be depressed.

She agrees. She suggests that I see my GP, that I might need something to help take the edge off whatever this is, and tells me that she wants to see me, to talk.

She asks me to tell my mother, and to get her to help tomorrow so that I can just take a backseat to everything. I tell her my husband is a great help. He is. He is like a rock and he is concerned and unsure about how to make this better. And I feel bad that I am this crying person who was his funny wife.

I need professional help. As I think those words to write them here I laugh hollowly.

I am going to get it. I am going to get through today and tomorrow, and hopefully in the future I won't remember my babies' baptism and think, 'I had postnatal depression then.' I hope I remember something nice about it.

I know I need help. I'm trying to get it.

I know that this will get better.

Depression is like a shit haircut. You know you won't always have a shit haircut but it takes time for it to grow out, so in the meantime you either wear a hat to conceal it completely or announce loudly, 'I AM AWARE I HAVE A SHIT HAIRCUT.'

Time to get some hair clips, I guess.

I send my mum the following text: 'I have postnatal depression. I keep crying randomly for no reason. I talked to my counsellor and she said that I did sound like I had depression and that I should talk to my GP on Monday. Not sure how tomorrow will go. I wish I was in a better place for it emotionally. I'm sorry.'

She calls me, she tells me that it's OK – this isn't the best time of year. She tells me tomorrow will be fine.

As my mother talks to me, my dad chimes in from the background, 'Did you know dads can get postnatal depression too?'

'Yes, Dad. Mum, is Dad just googling things?'

'Yes, he's talking to me as I'm talking to you.'

My dad then asks, 'What's postnatal drip?'

'Mum, he means postnasal drip. He's made a typo.'

Mum says, 'It's a nose thing.'

They want to help.

'Sure, we'll see you tomorrow!'

6 December

'Did you enjoy today?' Colm asked me after the baptism.

'I don't know,' I reply. 'I think so, it was fine.'

Today did go fine. I tell him that the bit I liked most was when we were seated in the church and each baby was quiet and happy, dressed in their baptism gown, being held by a grandmother. No one was asking how I was, and I didn't have to do anything but sit there in that moment.

When I am busy it is OK, it is hectic and I am able to do it. Having twins has possibly made me crazy-organized in certain regards, and today was no exception.

I had the odd moment when I thought I might cry – not because of anything in particular, just because the compulsion to do so came upon me. I find myself breathing through these moments, taking short, shallow breaths as if they are a contraction; something brief and compelling, part of some bigger thing. When I am alone the feeling comes back. I sense it in my abdomen, something large; as big as a decent-sized Christmas pudding. A ball of suppressed emotion. I feel it and I caress it with my mind; something hidden and unhealthy.

A friend said that crying with depression is like Hollywood crying: it's not an ugly thing, it is tears and grimacing. After I cry I ask Colm if it looks as if I've been crying. He says no, it looks as if I've forgotten to wear make-up or am tired.

I miss ugly crying, the kind where I sob and I am snotty, my face is red, blotchy and wet, and my chest is heaving with the force of the emotion being released. Afterwards I feel tired. I look as if I've been crying but I feel better, unburdened.

This depression has robbed me of that ability. My emotions once were a wondrous and complex beast, an ever-shifting swirl of colour and vibrancy, which I often couldn't contain or control.

Laughter that shook the heart of me, my ribcage sore from the joyous drawing-in of breath over and over, which left me feeling as if I would never be able to breathe again.

Sadness that crushed the heart in my chest like a can on the street, that aching pain that would clutch at my very being as I sobbed ugly tear after ugly tear.

Excitement that brushed on to fear and back again, thrilled and hopeful. Goosebumps forming on top of goosebumps, my skin electric and my stomach a rainforest of butterflies.

Now – right now – my emotions are simply

flashcards, a checklist of facial expressions and reactions.

The butterflies are dead.

My concern is this: today my children got baptized. And it was fine.

Our families were there, the babies were adorable and amazing – as they are – and this day passed me by.

And it was fine.

I did not, could not and cannot right now connect properly to the emotions that I should have felt.

I know what they should have been, as if reading a script with stage directions. I expressed them, but I did not really feel them.

And that is not fine.

I do not know if this is what depression is.

I do not want whatever it is.

Today, people took photos of the special occasion.

Tomorrow, I guess I will go and talk to the doctor.

I will talk to the doctor, I will talk to a counsellor and we will work on this.

My hope is that in time I will be able to look at today's photos and be able to feel the depth of emotion that I should have felt.

And that way the day won't be lost.

That way the day won't be just fine.

It will be better than fine because hopefully by then so will I.

7 December

Before, if ever something was wrong, the question 'How are you?' from someone I trusted would be my cue to cry.

Big, heavy sobs, and afterwards I might go to a bathroom and put on some make-up to make it look as if I hadn't been crying.

My doctor asks it.

I do not cry.

I just shake my head. I am not good.

'I think I have postnatal depression.'

It is normal, she tells me. I have two babies and there is a lot going on. We talk about it. I well up a little as I worry about being a bad parent, and that I'm messing up.

She tells me that as long as the babies are fed, warm and happy, they are fine. They don't realize that this is the best time for me to be depressed as they won't remember it. She tells me to have a routine. I assure her I do. I am regimented in the routine I have for the babies – it is their stability and maybe my own.

I am able to function for them but not for myself. Once they are asleep, my motivation abandons me. I just exist, not wanting to do anything other than just lie there in bed. Not doing anything.

She tells me I am not that bad. I am not in the blackness of black depression, I just need help getting back.

She gives me a prescription for antidepressants. I tell her I have never taken them before. She tells me I will probably be on them for four months and that they might take some time to start working.

I hug her as I leave. I don't feel the complete warmth of the hug but I feel it's something I would do – old me, anyways, and she is a good doctor.

In the pharmacy there's a backlog with prescriptions. Twenty minutes, I will have to wait. Twenty minutes for it to be filled. I go away and when I come back after twenty minutes it is still not done. I'm not annoyed – I don't feel much of anything. While I'm waiting, I pick up this giraffe toy called Sophie that I've heard people talking about and more teething powder for the babies. As I pay for all these items, the pharmacist talks to me about the tablets I now possess.

'Have you taken these before?'

'No.' I nod at the other purchases. 'I have postnatal depression.'

'Did your doctor say anything to you about starting on a half-dose for a week?'

'No.'

'Maybe ask her, as the side effects can be difficult.'

I tell her I will ask. We talk about my daughters and the fact that they are teething. She suggests other things – I already use them. I have a routine with the teething. It is part of my life now. I thank her and leave.

My counsellor sees me.

'How are you?' she asks.

I give a sigh and a half-shrug. 'Not good.'

Damn, I miss crying.

We talk about what is happening. I tell her about the lack of depth to my emotions, about going back to work and planning that.

She says some people with depression can't see a future for themselves.

When I tell her about how I feel, what I am telling her about is what I am not feeling. I feel stuck, as if there's something there that I am not reaching.

'It's like my mind went, "OK, you're having too many feelings right now so we're going to shut them down for a bit."'

'I wonder if the mind does that as a coping mechanism.'

'I was thinking about that last night and maybe it does. "You can get your feelings back later when you're ready for them."'

The thing is, during all of these interactions – with my doctor, the pharmacist, my counsellor – I am smiling.

Just because I'm depressed doesn't mean that I'm going around the place like Droopy the dog. Maybe a little in the breast department but I am smiling. I laugh lightly at things, I don't cry.

I tell my counsellor that I worry – as much as I can right now, which isn't a lot – that people won't believe that I'm depressed.

This isn't how depression is meant to look.

I am apathetic.

I am not sad.

I am not anything to any great degree.

She says this is why we need to work on this, why I need help and why I am getting it. She says that many people are clinically depressed, but they do not know it and they do not look for help.

God, I miss feeling 'self-congratulatory'.

On the bus home I read about the side effects of the medication. What I read makes me reluctant to take them. I don't feel *that* bad, do I need this? Do I need to take something for four months that has all these side effects?

Later, Colm and I put the babies, who are cranky with teething, down for a nap. Not before I let one of them chew on the toy giraffe I bought. I tell my husband she could be a lion when she grows up. After we put them to bed, we go for a nap ourselves in the spare room, both tired.

When we wake up I tell him about the tablets – about the side effects.

'When I got pregnant last year, I didn't think I'd be spending Christmas with nausea, vomiting and no energy, and then it would be the same again this Christmas. That's a bit shit. And apparently these tablets can take weeks to work. I just wanted something that would make me feel better straight away.'

'That's cocaine. You're thinking of cocaine. And you might not get the side effects. You're jumping ahead of yourself again, looking for the worst.'

'I thought maybe I didn't need to take them, that maybe I'd get better on my own. But the truth is, after we napped, you asked if I wanted to stay there because I wanted more sleep. I did want to stay there. But not because I wanted more sleep. Because I didn't want to get up. I just wanted to lie there and be nothing. This isn't me. I need to take those tablets, even though I don't want to.'

I say.

I do not cry.

I cannot cry.

9 December

Colm has a job offer. He says that I don't have to go back to work now, not as soon. I tell him I still want to go back. That I need to go back, that I can't keep going on like this. We need to arrange childcare. I need to email crèches and figure this out. Colm says he'll talk to his new job about starting part time for a month, to let the girls settle in.

11 December

I call into my work to tell them that I am coming back. I've already sent in the letter but I need to go in person. It feels surreal that I have children now, that I am depressed and they don't know, and that maybe I'll be depressed when I go back. I still don't know if I am making the right decision.

12 December

When I first started taking antidepressants I wasn't sure how they would make me feel. Sure, there were side effects: the yawning, nausea, feeling tired, then wondering if I felt tired because of the medication, the depression or the fact I've four-month-old twins.

I worried I would feel high, some sort of euphoria. Then I worried that I wasn't feeling better.

I also thought that the change would be instant, that things suddenly would be brighter – as if someone had opened the curtains in a dark room and chimed, 'Rise and shine, eh . . . depressed head, time to face the day.'

But that wasn't it.

Instead, I think I feel more like myself.

I know that's not euphoria, or me running around, singing, 'Let the sunshine in!' but it's something.

The weight in my chest has gone. It somehow slipped away while I was otherwise engaged. Although I haven't cried, I haven't really felt the need to.

I noticed today that I'm singing again. That's a weird tell to have – it makes me feel as if I'm a Disney princess or something – but when I'm happy I sing. In work I used to walk through the lab belting out various power ballads at people because I was happy. Today, I sang at the babies.

I made up this song when they were still in the womb.

The lyrics are simple: 'Babies, hmm mmmm hmm, babies, hmmm mmm.'

And then I would put in their names, our names.

After they were born I would sing it to keep them calm or if I was changing them, and my daughters used to coo along to it.

Today, I sang it to one of them and I meant it. It wasn't me just going through the motions and pretending that I'm not f**ked up, trying to push whatever joy my heart can contain to the front of the bleakness that clouded my mind.

I meant it.

And she smiled. She gave a small squeal of delight and shoved her hand in her mouth.

I know this is silly and this is small but it doesn't feel like a trick this time. It doesn't feel like one of those moments where I think I'm better but I'm not and the emptiness crowds back in.

I am feeling more like me.

That said, I'm going to continue taking the antidepressants until I'm told to stop, because I'm not going to say, 'Holy shit, I did this. I made me better!'

I will take them and I will talk to someone, because the depression came from somewhere and I need to close that door to stop it creeping back in.

13 December

The twins sat in high chairs for the first time today. Róisín didn't like it. She was tired and thought it was too high for her. Bronagh loved it. She loved getting fed in it more. After she ate all the baby rice, she kept throwing up her hands and squealing in victory.

Sure, we only decided at 2 a.m. this morning to start weaning them, because they keep waking up with hunger. Róisín eats like a lady – delicate mouthfuls, turning her head to one side softly if she's not interested. She's considered in her habits. Whereas Bronagh grabs your hand to get the food into her mouth as quickly as possible. She is super messy but loves every minute of it.

When she was in the womb she would go mental any time I ate. Now she's squealing through mouthfuls of baby rice and licking it off her bib. It's definite progress from our last attempt at baby rice. We should all be more Bronagh.

ENTERTAINING BABIES

Beyond the realm of feeding, changing, and keeping babies warm and safe is the realm of entertaining them. Luckily, a huge range of toys has been made to assist parents in this.

My parents got the kids a toy. It's a plastic horse that talks and plays music.

Colm hates it.

'I don't think I've ever hated anything as much as that horse.'

The babies bat the horse.

It asks, 'Can I have a carrot?'

'I think we have some in the bin. I'll help you find them,' Colm replies.

One of the ideas I had before becoming a parent was that we wouldn't have any toys that made annoying noises, but that idea was abandoned and I've made a helpful flowchart to explain why.

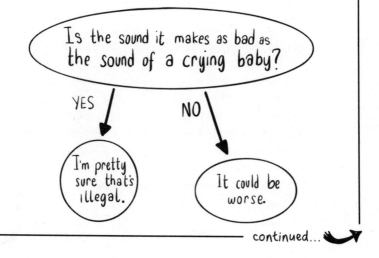

"I saw a toy but it makes noise.

Should I buy it or will it annoy me?"

Is the sound it makes as bad as the sound of a crying baby?

YES → I'm pretty sure that's illegal.

NO → It could be worse.

continued...

In fact, most baby toys are sold on the premise that they somehow stimulate the brain of your child and turn them into some kind of baby genius, which alleviates the guilt of buying them something to entertain them.

WHAT TOY ADVERTS SAY

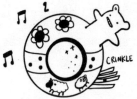

High contrast colours.
Multiple stimulating textures.
Improves hand-eye co-ordination.

WHAT TOY ADVERTS SHOULD SAY

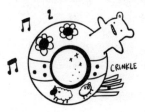

Distracts them for at least five minutes!

YOU COULD HAVE A COFFEE!

That said, most of the time the babies want things to play with that aren't toys.

Some babies have a comfort toy – sometimes called a transitional object – which is something they use to help when self-comforting. One of my daughters has a monkey. It's called Monkey because it's hard to be creative on four hours' sleep. She loves Monkey. I have no idea where Monkey was made or by whom, and I will never be able to buy a replacement, which brings me to the graph opposite.

continued...

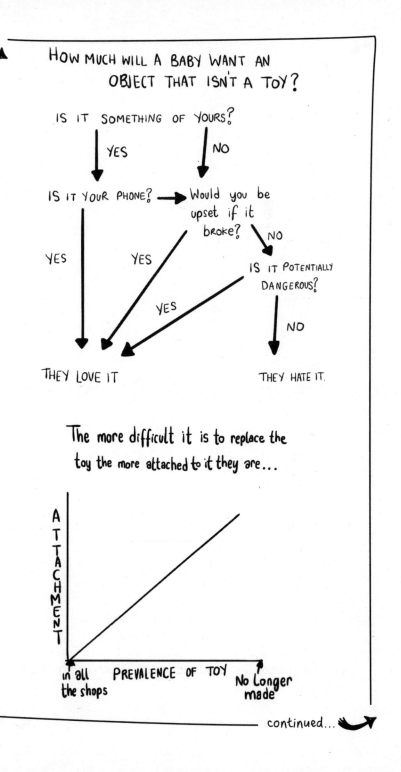

continued...

This issue is so real that a number of eBay accounts are doing quite well by charging unreasonable sums for replacement comfort toys, because how much would you pay for a decent night's sleep? I couldn't run a business like that because knowing my luck my kids would become attached to all of the objects and I'd never be able to sell them or rid my house of them.

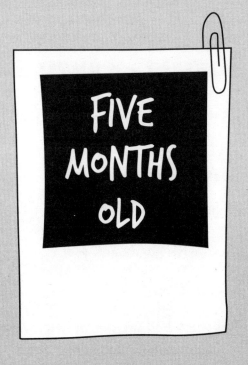

16 DECEMBER – 15 JANUARY 2016

* Reacts and turns towards sounds
  and voices

* Grasps smaller objects

* Rolls over in both directions

* Plays with hands and feet

* Begins 'creeping'

* Supports bodyweight on legs when held
  in standing position

* Reaches with one hand

* Transfers objects from hand to hand

16 December

Weaning discovery of the day: the cat likes baby rice and will eat that stuff off the floor. We haven't asked her to clean the children, as I doubt they would have any skin left by the time she was finished with them.

18 December

Róisín's eating technique involves diving at the spoon in my hand. Bronagh's involves rubbing the food all over herself and absorbing the nutrients through her skin.

21 December

When on the phone, a crying baby is the new 'I'm going into a tunnel, gotta go!'

Today I went to scope out a crèche. Colm and I decided on it because it's near our house and I haven't heard any reports in the news that the children there are hit regularly with red-hot pokers.

I go on my own and the receptionist wonders that I might have brought the babies. I lie and say they're being fed, but the fact is I haven't brought them because I don't want them to know what I'm contemplating doing.

'How old will the babies be?' asks the receptionist.

'Almost six months.'

'A lot of people wait until ten months,' she says casually.

'YOU ARE THE WORST MOTHER IN THE WORLD!' a voice in my head shouts.

The manager shows me around the place. There's a baby room, which has a number of babies in it (so no lies there) and three staff. I'm told how the babies are fed, about routines, and when they get naps. There's a list of instructions for each child.

The room looks 'lived in'. I'm sure it was bright at

some stage but it has been pawed by a number of small hands – all of the rooms have been. It's probably a good thing – it shows that they haven't had to scrub any blood off the walls.

The feeling that I am making a terrible mistake haunts me for the rest of the tour. I am shown various other rooms containing children at different stages of development – sitting babies, wobbling tweenies, running toddlers. I ask the manager which is her favourite room.

'The tweenies room is the hardest. They're just starting to walk, they get frustrated easily and they bite one another, but it's nice to see them take their first steps and hear their first words.'

YOU ARE THE WORST MOTHER IN THE WORLD. A STRANGER IS GOING TO SEE YOUR BABIES' FIRST STEPS AND HEAR THEIR FIRST WORDS.

I want to ask her if I am doing the right thing.

I don't feel like I am. I feel like I'm weak, selfish, and that I should be better at this mothering thing. That I am handing over my responsibilities to strangers for money. The cost of childcare, five days a week for the two babies, will work out to be €1,715 a month.

A figure that is absolutely insane.

As I'm leaving, the receptionist asks if I want to confirm the places.

I say I am unsure – I need to talk to my husband.

NO, I DON'T WANT THEM HERE! THIS IS INSANE! WHY AM I DOING THIS?!

'I need to talk to my husband,' I repeat.

Sheepishly, I take the information sheets she gives me and a form to fill out.

I leave, dazed.

I go home to Colm and I cry.

'I've read it's normal for parents to cry the first time they leave the crèche,' he says.

I think that probably means the first time that parents leave their babies there, but I don't say it.

My five-month-old identical girls are teething. Until now, the biggest symptom was them chewing their fists in every goddamn photo.

Apparently, nothing in this world tastes better than baby hands. They even chew each other's for a bit of variety.

That was fine, but now the drooling has resulted in a rash on their chins.

What can I put on that?

Right now they look as if we decided to shave their faces for Christmas.

At this stage it's probably not a bad thing if I let them cover their rashy chins with their delicious fists.

24 December

It is our first Christmas together as a family.

The babies do not know what Christmas is. They don't understand the concept of presents either – mostly because they believe that all objects somehow belong to them. They do not know who Santa is, or that we might be hiding his true identity.

When we become new parents, we find ourselves reconnecting with Santa after many years, like an old school friend we've found on Facebook. On Christmas Eve I chant, 'Santa! Santa! Santa!' I'm giddy with the excitement and the secrecy of it all.

Tomorrow is the twins' first Christmas, but they think it's any other Friday. Just kidding – they've no idea what Friday is.

25 December

'Happy Christmas, babies!' we say.

It's Christmas! The babies are up early – just like every other day – but today Santa has been. Maybe

Santa has always been. Colm and I are very excited. The girls are somehow always excited. We give them presents to unwrap – they bat them with their hands and there is dissatisfied shouting because essentially we have just put a ball of paper on top of them.

'We should unwrap the presents,' I say to Colm.

And we start carefully unwrapping them.

'Shouldn't we rip them open so they can see how it's meant to be done?' suggests Colm.

So we do, and in true Christmas baby fashion, they ditch the presents and play with the wrapping paper. Then, after about five minutes, want us to take it away.

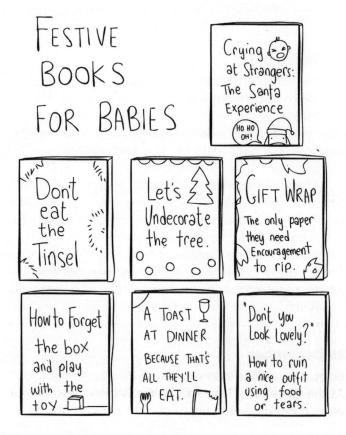

Christmas together has made me realize that every family's Christmas is a hodgepodge of tradition and 'how do you spend a day all by yourselves?' Our Christmas is an amalgamation of Colm's family traditions (a fry-up for breakfast and eating dinner in the evening) and my family tradition of drinking Shloer with dinner and having sausagemeat stuffing.

However, Colm and I have our own traditions too. One that we've had for a few years is a bat glove puppet, with its wings outstretched, on top of our Christmas tree. We couldn't find a star.

27 December

Me: 'You look tired. You need to sleep!'
Babies: [*cranky crying and wriggling*]
Me: 'Go to sleep. You're sleepy!'
Babies: [*shouting and more crying*]
Me: 'Calm down and go to sleep.'

I pull blankets over them and they drift off. Being a parent is a bit like being a really stern hypnotist.

28 December

A flaw of the human mind is that it finds it hard to stay in the present.

We drift back to the past constantly – remembering and reliving – and into an unknowable future, trying to imagine scenarios and how we will feel in them.

When I look at the children – who, I am aware, aren't even six months old – I am remembering how small they used to be. Their tiny hands, their small hiccuping faces, how I'd support their chin with two fingers so they could drink a bottle because they couldn't lift their heads up. At the same time, I say things like, 'When they're older we can bring them to the zoo and they'll know the names of the animals but not be assholes about it.' Or, 'One day they will tell me they hate me.'

Being a parent has made me think about my relationship with my own parents. For me, my parents have been a constant, more or less. They have always been adults and have always looked the same. Although I know this isn't true – of course they have looked different. My father used to have huge sideburns and a hook for a hand, and my mother had a perm for a time, I think. Unless I'm just assuming that every woman in the eighties had a perm.

Which could be true.

However, when I think of them, I don't see them as having changed.

Over the years there have been moments when I've realized that my parents are getting older. A heart attack, a fall, cataracts – frailties that come with age. The small things that remind you that your parents are human, because you forget.

It took me a long time – longer than it should have – to see that my parents were fallible adults trying to be infallible, because that's what children need.

For years and years – probably until I was in my late twenties – it felt as if my parents treated me like a child, which deepened a frustration in me and created a rift between us. There were angry phone calls and tears. I wanted them to treat me like an adult, to let me grow in their eyes.

Maybe after years of trying to be infallible it is difficult to let that mask drop, to be questioned, disobeyed, to realize that your time actively parenting is over.

Now I am a parent, I wonder what my parents see when they look at me. Do they see the baby, all gummy smiles, trying to crawl, being washed in a sink? The small girl holding on to her father's legs, standing on his feet as he walks, laughing? The curly-haired girl fighting with her brother on the sitting-room carpet, carrying her

UNCONDITIONAL LOVE...

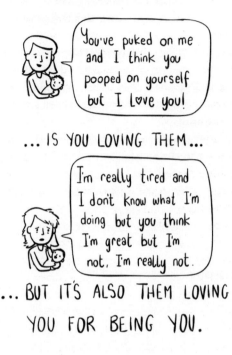

... IS YOU LOVING THEM...

... BUT IT'S ALSO THEM LOVING
YOU FOR BEING YOU.

teddies around the house, sleeping in front of the fire with the dog? The young girl on her first day at school, crying in the classroom, crying at the kitchen table, saying that the girls at school called her fat? Showing them something she drew, wanting them to be proud? Reading at night even when they told her to turn off the light? A teenager, laughing and telling dirty jokes? Being told she has cancer – she is only fifteen? Her going to college? Her with her first boyfriend, the other boyfriends? Seeing her less and less? Her as a wife, then as a mother?

For me, my parents wear one face when I think of them. That image, an amalgam of who they are, is cast in my mind.

They have changed so little in my eyes.

Yet I've grown up, completely. They knew me before I came into this world and watched the years pour into my development.

Now I'm an adult, but when they look at me I can imagine they may see every incarnation of me at once – an image shifting back and forth, so many faces and ages that it must be hard for them to hold me in their mind as me in the present.

To my own children, I may become the rarely changing person, infallible and constant, and years from now they may realize that I am human, flawed and fragile.

And I might wonder where my babies went to.

But right now, I still have moments when I wonder if I'm grown up enough to have kids.

31 December

Happy New Year

I'm celebrating it with the cat! Just kidding! The cat already made plans.

Don't wait up

Last New Year's Eve I drew the cartoon on the previous page, but I did in fact spend it with the cat, eating crackers because I was nauseous.

Very few people knew I was pregnant at that point.

Or that I was pregnant with twins.

It was a fairly miserable New Year's Eve.

This New Year I've two babies. I have two babies.

Me.

Well, us.

Colm and I, not myself and the cat.

Conclusion: last New Year's Eve was spent feeling very tired, lonely and sick.

This New Year's Eve I can eat food! Colm is here and I've made people come out my fanny in the intervening year! Two of them! They are in bed because they don't feel any social pressure to enjoy tonight.

And I could still vomit if I fancied a bit of nostalgia.

I don't.

Happy New Year.

1 January 2016

I had my first stress dream last night about going back to work.

I hate dreams like that. I think I should get paid overtime if I'm spending extra hours in work – even if it's in my head.

4 January

Colm starts his new job tomorrow so today I took the babies to the crèche to see how they'd get on.

It's a brave new world.

To be honest, it's a bit crap. I love my kids. I'm not looking forward to going back to work but I have to. Also, from a financial point of view, childcare is like getting a bag of money and f**king it on to a fire.

I could put this all off and off but it won't make it easier or anyone happier.

Meanwhile, various websites and national newspapers are referring to me today as 'an illustrator'. They're praising what I've created – a cartoon about being afraid to go back to work.

Funny, that – I am afraid to go back to work.

But.

I'm not an illustrator.

I don't get paid for that.

I can't pay my rent with that.

I'm a scientist.

I'm a disillusioned scientist who finds life bloody challenging at times.

5 January

I've brought the babies to crèche again to settle in for an hour.

They look so little.

All the other babies are monsters compared to them.

I'm going to have to give them knives to defend themselves.

6 January

The girls spent a settling-in hour without me in the crèche today. It was odd leaving them in there. A little emotional for me at the start, but I went back and, seriously, it was as if they hadn't realized I'd left.

The women in the crèche were super excited about having these identical babies to play with and I had to teach them how to tell them apart.

One of the women loves Bronagh. Today, when I got her back, she smelled of this woman's perfume. I kissed my baby and she smelled like someone else. That felt odd.

When I'm at home I do weird things with the babies

and sing at them and I'm silly. It's hard to think about other people doing those things with my kids.

I really like doing accents for them, and Bronagh loves it. To make her laugh I do this silly Russian voice: 'Oooh, I am Bronagh. I like milk-milk, it is delish-e-ous. The milk of the people, the milk-milk for all.'

She laughs and she smiles and she thinks it is great.

Now there is this other woman who loves Bronagh and who Bronagh keeps smiling at . . . stealing her affection.

Then I realize something.

This. Woman. Is. Lithuanian.

As far as Bronagh is concerned, this person does the hilarious accent all day.

She must think it's amazing.

She must never know.

7 January

The girls are in crèche for two hours today.

This gives me babyless time.

I've decided to have lunch.

Outside.

Alone.

I mean, in a café. I'm not eating bread out of a bag outside the crèche in the rain, steaming up the window with my breath.

9 January

My parents are visiting.

My dad said, 'I could hardly sleep last night I was so excited about seeing the girls!'

'And me?'

'Yes, you too,' he says, holding on to a baby while making faces at the other one.

My parents are looking after the babies while Colm and I go to a restaurant for lunch.

The waiter asks Colm if he would like a drink.

He says, 'OH, GOD, YES!'

What he didn't realize he was doing was making it look as if I was the worst date in the world.

The waiter looked at me with pity for the entire meal.

10 January

I told the babies that I'm going back to work tomorrow.

They had no idea.

They didn't even know I had a job.

11 January

I am back in work. It feels as if I never left – as if I just went on a short holiday and came back – but it's different. John – with whom I shared a workspace – he's gone. He left for another job before I even had the babies. The other girls who fell pregnant in the great everyone-is-pregnant-at-the-same-time rush aren't here either – they're on maternity leave. The office feels a bit empty, I feel a bit out of place, but I'm back.

One advantage of being in work: I can go to the toilet and have a poo in peace.

And get paid for the pleasure.

'Do you have separation anxiety?' someone asked me this morning.

I scoffed. The notion is ridiculous. I'd only just left the babies and I'll be seeing them again later.

After lunch, I work on an experiment I've done so often I can do it without thinking.

Instead, I think of them.

I have left them.

I am here now without them.

My rational mind is thrown out the window in a mess of emotion and longing.

I miss them so much it physically hurts.

'I miss my kids, I miss my kids, I miss my kids.'

I say it over and over in my head as I work in my lab coat, and my gloves, with my Petri dishes.

I feel it, but I don't let it show.

Someone distracts me and I am grateful for it.

I am counting down the minutes until I can go home, because I love them.

I love my kids.

12 January

The babies are spending their first full day in crèche. Yesterday Colm was looking after them; today, women I barely know.

At lunchtime someone asked me if the girls were in crèche. They themselves had children in crèche, and they asked if I had phoned to see how the twins were getting on.

I hadn't realized I could do this.

Immediately, I felt guilty for not knowing this was an option, yet thrilled that it was.

I called and the receptionist went to enquire. She said they were being model pupils (it's not a school) and they were doing great. She didn't put them on the phone, or hold the phone near enough so I could shout, 'MAMMY MISSES YOU!'

Because I did miss them.

I told someone at work that I had to leave to pick up my kids.

She said it sounded strange. She's known me for five years and suddenly I'm someone who goes to pick up their kids.

Was I excited about the idea of picking up my kids? Yes.

Very much so. Our arrangement is that Colm drops them off in the morning and I collect them.

I've just got on the bus when Colm sends me a text saying, 'GO RESCUE THE BABIES!' but I'm already on my way.

In the crèche, I have to find our buggy and figure out how to unfold it. Then I go into the baby room. The baby wardens inform me how the girls' day went, what they ate, when they slept – riveting stuff, really. One of them points out that Bronagh has a tooth erupting. I tell them I know.

I realize that I will have to inspect my children each and every morning for differences to avoid a 'Surprise! Your child is changing and you're missing the majority of it!' moment. I'm sure there will be plenty of these in future.

As we are leaving, I ask the Lithuanian baby warden what her name is.

She tells me.

I make sure I am pronouncing it correctly.

And then I promptly forget it.

Now I've to get Colm to ask her.

When I get the babies back home the house is cold. They are in the buggy and after I put the heating on, I sing to them and they both coo excitedly. I sing our song. I guess they're doing the baby equivalent of 'CHOOOOOON!'

I cuddle the babies and notice they smell of perfume again. I think it belongs to the baby warden whose name I forget. I don't like this – they don't smell like babies, they smell like whores.

Kidding, but I worry that not only do I now miss their smell but that I also associate that perfume – whatever it is – with my kids. I further worry that maybe they're spraying the babies with perfume to make me think they've been cuddled all day when in fact they've been in a bin.

I played with the girls for about forty-five minutes. Bronagh squealed, blew bubbles and made noises in an effort to tell me that they *had* put her in a bin, but I just thought she was being cute and blew bubbles back.

I felt an incredible pressure to make these babies feel as loved by me as they could be in the brief window between crèche and bedtime, a rising guilt that maybe I'm doing the wrong thing, that they will hold it against me, that I'm not there to share their lives.

They went to bed overly tired.

I am incredibly tired myself. As physically draining as looking after babies is, I've forgotten how mentally taxing my work is, as well as running round a lab.

My hope is that I will get used to it after a while.

Right now, I need a quick nap before I crack on with everything that needs doing before I can go to bed myself.

SO ENDS THEIR FIRST DAY IN BABY PRISON!

GOING BACK TO WORK

Motherhood: that weird gap on your LinkedIn profile that will have future employers raising their eyebrows.

Why not fill it in by being liberal with the truth?

'I worked in the dairy production industry.'

'I was R&D manager for a manufacturing project. We made two prototypes, spent months trying to iron out the kinks before we decided that we didn't want to go into mass production.'

'I was in charge of training new employees to defecate in a toilet rather than in their pants.'

'I spent two years studying human developmental behaviours.'

'I was in charge of a small office with two employees. Despite a number of written and verbal warnings about putting office equipment in their mouths we had to let them go.'

ᘓᘓᘓᘓᘓᘓᘓ

continued... ➤

Whenever I used to think about working mothers I'd imagine these powerful career women for whom having a baby wasn't even their focus – they gave birth then went straight back to their work. In my mind, these women were always power-dressed and straight from the 1980s, but that wasn't me.

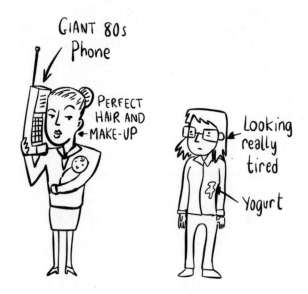

GIANT 80s Phone

PERFECT HAIR AND MAKE-UP

Looking really tired

Yogurt

For me, going back to work was like when a character in a book or a film returns to their normal life at the end of an amazing adventure. Although they feel changed, things haven't changed for anyone else. It was a bit like at the end of *The Lord of the Rings* when all the hobbits go back to their lives in the Shire.

The person who was covering my maternity leave was still there. It must be difficult to be given a job on the basis that someone has left to have a baby, with the added uncertainty of whether they may or may not come back. She was still doing my job, though. I knew *I* should probably be doing my job but no one really told me what was going on.

continued...

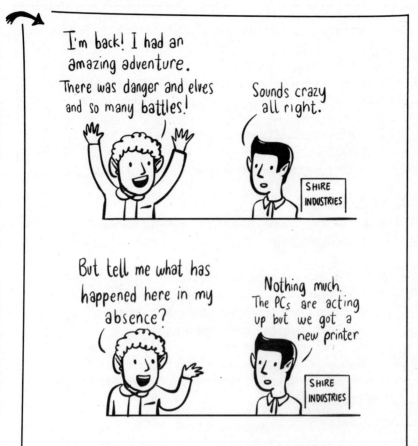

As grateful as I was to have been entitled to maternity leave, on my return I felt as if I almost had to compete for a job I had been doing for years, simply because the situation could have been handled better.

I'm aware that some people believe that once a woman decides to have children then she no longer cares about her career. However, if anything, I needed to justify the time I wasn't spending with my kids. If anything, when I was at work, I was actually more productive than ever, because I'd spent the past six months working non-stop. The other benefits to being back at work were being able to drink coffee while it was still hot, and having regular adult conversations that

— continued... ➥

weren't the result of me being overly friendly in a shop.

I've also become part of an unofficial club of working parents, distinguishable because we're all very tired and because we have small conversations about the activities of our children that are contributing to our tiredness. The other thing we have in common is the fact that at the end of the day we have to go to collect our kids.

13 January

11.10 a.m. Our landlord wants to sell our house. FANTASTIC TIMING!

6.40 p.m. How can life get better?
Vomiting and diarrhoea, that's how.
But don't worry, I'm the only one with it.
Ah, bathroom bin, we meet again.

An advantage to having babies is the increased number of receptacles around the house into which I can throw up. Case in point, the baby bath. Then, later, the nappy bin.

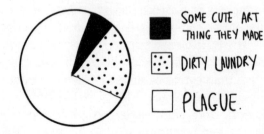

THINGS MY KIDS BRING HOME FROM CHILDCARE.

SOME CUTE ART THING THEY MADE

DIRTY LAUNDRY

PLAGUE.

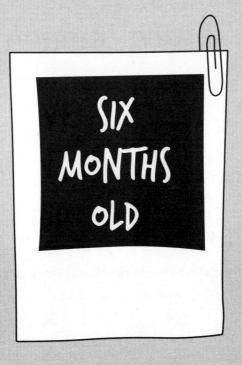

16 JANUARY - 15 FEBRUARY

* Imitates sounds

* Begins eating solid foods

* Sits without support

* Picks up dropped objects

* Sits in high chair

* May start teething (this can occur
  from 4-7 months of age)

* Enjoys hearing own voice

* Vocalizes to mirror and toys

* Begins to make sounds that resemble
  one-syllable words

16 January

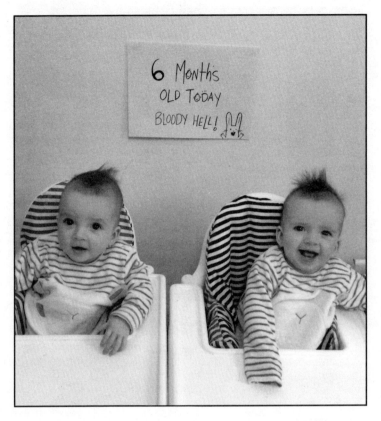

Bloody hell!
We made it this far.

18 January

Parenting quotes from Colm this weekend:
'Why do they keep kicking me in the balls?'
'They pull my beard every time they're near my face. Like, really pull it.'
'I'm exhausted. Could I not just nip up to a hotel for the night?'

19 January

Today's baby discovery: when babies have a cough and they hack up a big greener, at no point does it occur to them not to swallow it.

And there is no way to persuade them to spit it out.

Both of you just live with the knowledge of what's going on.

Them thinking there isn't a choice.

You thinking they're making the wrong one.

And when they puke all the gobbers up on to your jumper, your name is Colm and you say, 'Why do the babies always puke on me and not you?'

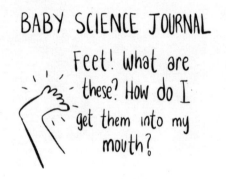

BABY SCIENCE JOURNAL

Feet! What are these? How do I get them into my mouth?

21 January

I've discovered that having kids means that people with kids ask me about them, and I ask about their kids.

A benefit of having twins: getting to say 'I HAVE KIDS' makes me sound as if I've been doing this parenting stuff for years.

23 January

My parents come to visit. While they are here I trim the babies' nails and I manage to take a bit of Róisín's fingertip. The tiniest bit of skin.

She then bleeds for ages, covering her dress, my mum and the playmat in dabs of blood.

'Don't put a plaster on, in case she chokes on it,' my mum says.

Then we try various ways to make the bleeding stop before putting a massive plaster on the cut.

'I am not abusing my children,' I say to my mother as we wipe blood off things.

The entire time Róisín could not give a f**k that one of her fingers has basically been turned into a serial killer's bingo marker.

I am not winning at parenting today.

25 January

At six months old the babies now have teeth – two small teeth each. They use them to bite things – mostly their hands, my fingers, people's chins – all with no actual objective other than to test them out.

Colm and I are feeding them mush. Sometimes I give them something to chew that is solid food, such as a banana, but all they do is just make it wet and bits of it fall off. If they aren't trying to push the food in with their fists, they are trying to grab the spoon and 'help'.

In fact, they keep using their newfound limb control to 'help' in other ways.

They are not helping.

A baby trying to feed itself a babygro with poop stains on it as you change their nappy is not helping either. It is the opposite of helping.

So far this week they have both had colds, which basically involved them hacking away like someone who's smoked sixty a day for twenty years. They know that they are coughing up phlegm, and they think that they just swallow it. It's either leave them to it or use a nasal aspirator – the hose for the nose – to suck snot out of their nostrils. They do not like this thing. They protest and use their barely competent hands to push me away.

Part of the weekend was spent dealing with baby diarrhoea. This involved changing nappies a lot, and poo seeping out of the nappies and on to their babygros.

When they are sick I worry that I made them sick, and I know I have to make them better. The reality is, babies get minor illnesses, but when they do it's a new experience for them. It must be terrifying. Maybe they think it's normal, that it's a new part of their life and it will always be this way as they grumble and are dosed up with Calpol, the world's stickiest substance.

Paracetamol syrup doesn't taste great, but they like it because it is sweet and comes out of a tube into their sore mouths and they have the option to allow part of it to leak on to and stain whatever duvet cover they are currently lying on. At least they now recognize 'the purple wand' and are able and willing to swallow (at least some of) the medicine.

Baby diarrhoea was fine until it was accompanied by vomiting and the worry that they would dehydrate, which resulted in me trying to get hold of a GP on a Sunday. Luckily, a friend is a doctor and gave me advice because I was having one of those rare 'What the f**k do I do now?' moments. Turns out we should resort to using a syringe to get fluids into their mouths. During this palaver they were in good form, smiling.

'Stop smiling. This is serious.'

Not a single f**k given.

Sick babies are hard work. According to Colm, 'Two sick babies is like having six healthy babies.'

If I had six babies I'd definitely attach them all to a sled as soon as they could crawl.

'MUSH! MUSH!' I'd then say (as I ordered their breakfast).

27 January

The best part of my day is picking up my kids from the crèche and giving the finger to all the crèche workers while shouting, 'I'M THEIR MUM! Me! Not you! You're NOTHING!'

Just kidding, but I love picking them up.

2 February

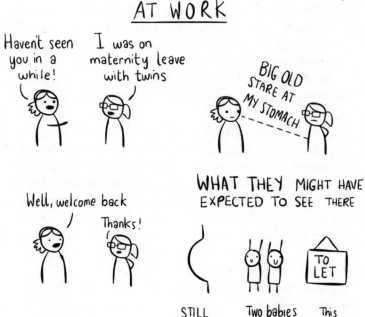

AT WORK

Haven't seen you in a while!

I was on maternity leave with twins

BIG OLD STARE AT MY STOMACH

Well, welcome back

Thanks!

WHAT THEY MIGHT HAVE EXPECTED TO SEE THERE

STILL PREGNANT!

Two babies hanging off me.

TO LET

This sign!

4 February

Last night Colm and I talked about getting our shit together.

I cried.

I cried because sometimes it feels as if we will never

175

find a new house. I'm OK with renting but not when we are being forced to move. Our current landlord wants to sell this house we're in – we moved in when our previous landlord wanted to sell that house. This might give the impression that we're bad tenants but it's not that, this is just what's happening right now in Dublin. There are fewer houses to rent as it's easier to sell a house to make a profit than to keep it and tenants. It's an awful position to be in when you have babies who need parents with their shit together to make them feel stable and safe.

After I cried, I told Colm that we don't have to have everything sorted straight away.

I was telling him but I was really telling myself.

Being an adult is hard.

Until I had kids I used to feel as if I was letting my parents down. Now I feel like I'm letting the kids down instead.

When I was younger I thought that being an adult would be all staying up late and eating the nice biscuits.

And it is!

But as you're eating the biscuits you're worrying about getting your shit together and not really enjoying the biscuits.

5 February

This morning, as I was holding Bronagh, she got a bit sick on me.

'Quick, Colm, hand me the baby wipes!'

As he reaches for them, Róisín, who he is holding, throws up all over him.

'Well, the baby wipes are mine now.'

Two baby funsies!

Róisín's diarrhoea and vomiting got to the point where I couldn't get her to keep any fluids down, so we're now in the children's hospital.

It's 7 p.m. and we've been here since 4 p.m. Because we've two babies Colm is home with Bronagh.

I'm given some oral rehydration solution mixed with orange cordial to try to give her while we wait. She's not a fan.

She might be improving because she spent ages attempting to get the attention of a three-year-old boy.

He was terrified when she giggled at him.

She's not improving, she just pooped herself again. Some day off this is.

So we are home, after almost four hours in the hospital.

Róisín started to keep fluids down, which I was having to syringe into her every ten minutes or so. She then decided to smile at the doctor, pretending she was fine, BUT SHE WAS BETRAYED BY THE POOP IN HER NAPPY.

He told me I had done everything right, which is good, and is the opposite of 'We have to take your children away.' I asked about managing it better and he gave me advice and some anti-sickness meds for Róisín. To help her keep her shit together. Literally.

Oddly, that was the longest amount of time I've spent with Róisín on her own. It was nice in the strangest way, because my attention is usually divided constantly between two babies. In future I will try to have more alone time with one baby and Colm can take the other.

6 February

Ever wonder exactly how many loads of washing your machine can do in a day? Why not push it to its limit by simply having six-month-old twins with vomiting and diarrhoea?

Ever think that maybe you have too many sleepsuits and baby blankets? You don't now, they're all covered in puke and poop, and are currently wearing out your washing machine.

Some other observations from the frontline of caring for a baby with D&V:

- Marvel at the fact that your daughter keeps projectile vomiting down your husband.
- Suggest that maybe he wear something which is easier to clean, because you're sick of washing his dressing gown.
- Enjoy waiting in Temple Street's emergency department on your own with the twin who is most sick, constantly apologizing for the room taken up by the double buggy, and assuring people that she is a twin.
- Don't say, 'I'm not lying! There are two of them!'
- Struggle to use the syringe you've been given to give your baby fluids. She doesn't cry but does manage to poo herself twice in the waiting room.
- Have someone in the waiting room tell you about how she breastfed all her children until they were eight months old.
- Consider suggesting that maybe she should get some sort of medal.
- Watch as your seemingly well baby laughs at the doctor, who you see after almost four hours. Assure him that she is sick, then realize it's OK – he'll believe you – as she's just pooped herself again.
- Be told that she is OK and that you are doing the right thing.
- Almost cry with relief that she's all right while walking the both of you home.
- Eat things full of sugar because you're so tired.
- Try to sleep.
- Get up and battle puke, poop and laundry again with your husband.
- Realize that even though a baby can have done the biggest poop in the world, because she's laughing as you change her she will still look as cute as hell.
- Wonder which side of the family she got that from.

8 February

I've started to notice that mothers with babies act differently, depending on whether or not I have my babies with me.

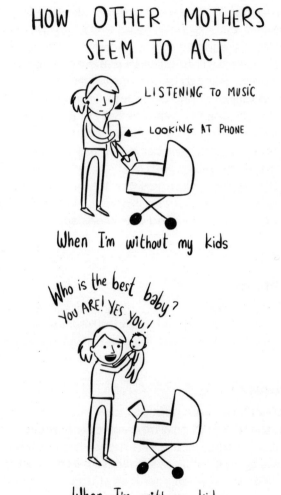

HOW OTHER MOTHERS SEEM TO ACT

LISTENING TO MUSIC

LOOKING AT PHONE

When I'm without my kids

Who is the best baby? YOU ARE! YES YOU!

When I'm with my kids

One time, I was changing one of the twins and another mother came into the changing room. I started fussing over my baby and I couldn't help but wonder why I was doing this. It struck me that there's an unspoken paranoia that if you slip up as a parent in front of another parent, they might report you to a secret parenting organization for being unfit. I call this feeling 'fear of being reported by the secret parenting police'.

The secret parenting police could be anyone, but they are most likely to be other mothers, which is why I find myself acting differently around them. I feel that I have to look like I know what I'm doing and that whatever I'm doing I'm enjoying it, all of it. In return, other mothers alter their behaviour around me, but only when I have my babies with me.

That's because when you don't have your kids with you, you may or may not be a parent. You could just be someone who is really tired and keeps spilling yogurt on herself.

10 February

I gave Róisín a rusk.

She held it up in the air with both hands.

Colm asked her, 'What are you doing? Saying mass?'

14 February

The babies have been going to the crèche for over a month now. I didn't know how any of this would work out, but it's working. Sure, this month has contained an insane amount of illness. If illness had a Christmas, I think it would be 'when your kids start in childcare'.

At best, when sending them there I hoped that my kids would be looked after until I could rescue them in the evening, and they are. However, I wasn't expecting that they would be loved. The staff love my kids and

I love them for that. When I collect the babies, the crèche workers help me get them ready to bring them home. Sometimes it's the girls in the baby room and sometimes it's Jean on reception.

I like Jean. She has a dry sense of humour and she's the person who tells me how the girls are if I call, or calls if the girls aren't well. She also tells me how much she enjoys going out at the weekend with the wicked glee of someone who has already raised her kids. These people have become adult conversation in my life. Sure, we talk about the kids, but if picking up my kids is a highlight of my day, then the people there are highlights of my day too.

Today it is Valentine's Day, so I made the crèche a card from my kids (also from me and Colm) and bought them a box of chocolates. My babies made me a Valentine's card too, using their feet, which explains the red paint on their soles last night that I initially thought was yet another illness.

WAYS TO AVOID BEING REPORTED BY THE SECRET PARENTING POLICE

1. When another mother approaches, you must fuss over your baby like you have never fussed before.
2. If asked, tell them you are still breastfeeding. Even if you aren't asked, try to drop it into conversation.
3. Give parenting advice, even if unsolicited. Showing that you know something about what you are doing will definitely make them think you aren't just making it up as you go along.
4. If another parent posts a photo of their child online, try to point out at least one dangerous object in the photo, even if that item is 10 metres away and the baby is unable even to lift its own head.
5. In all social-media posts, only say positive things about motherhood and, ideally, embellish them with a hashtag such as #blessed.

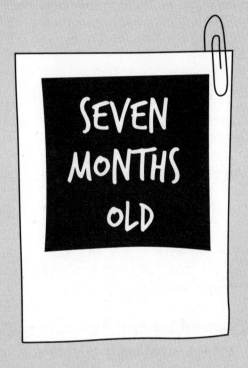

16 FEBRUARY – 15 MARCH

* Responds to name

* Uses voice to express joy and displeasure

* Finds objects that are partially hidden

* Explores with hands and mouth

* Drags objects towards self

* May start crawling (this can occur
     from 6-10 months of age)

* Jabbers and combines syllables

* Enjoys social play

16 February

The babies are seven months old now. Look at them attempting to eat everything on this earth by slowly gumming it until it softens and falls to the mercy of their two teeth.

Bronagh can kind of sit up now. Róisín can too, but falls forward slowly, like a drunk trying to keep his shit together at a bar. They can sort of move if you put them down to crawl – not proper crawling, but they'd definitely lose a game of musical statues.

IF SCIENTISTS WERE BABIES

Our research must discover a new element.

And what will we do when we find it?

SHOVE IT IN OUR MOUTHS!

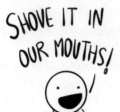

Until the funding body takes it off us!

20 February

The babies have become obsessed with my necklace. The necklace that is essentially my engagement ring.

Whenever I hold them they look at me, smile, look down, notice the necklace, get this crazy look on their faces and lunge for it. Their obsession with it has gone *Lord of the Rings*. I've even started doing a Gollum impression of their efforts: 'We wants it, my precious, we needs it! Stupid, fat Mammy! Gives it to us!'

I actually took it off to stop them clawing my neck with their tiny bird-like nails, before realizing that it was the only thing distracting them from grabbing my glasses. They're essentially magpies. Colm doesn't have a necklace so they go for his eyes.

Earlier today, they were sitting side by side and I dangled the necklace for them. They wanted it, it was now free from my neck, grabbable and, most importantly, they could finally gum it.

Róisín was a bit better at reaching for it. Smiling, she would hold it, look at my hand to tell me she wanted me to let go of the chain, which I wouldn't, so she'd then stuff the necklace in her mouth. Unfortunately, any time Róisín had the chain, Bronagh would get angry. She wanted the necklace too – she wasn't sure why but she wanted it. I gave it to her. Like Róisín, she'd get annoyed that I was holding the chain. I gave in and let go. Finally it was all hers – for the whole ten seconds it took Róisín to grab it and yank it away from her.

This is a small thing, but it's the first time they've shown possessiveness over an object, which – let's be clear here – is *my* bloody object.

By the way, the times I gave Bronagh the necklace and Róisín kept yanking it away, I did laugh. Something which did not go down well in Bronagh camp. Neither did the Gollum impressions.

Still, they're growing up fast. They'll be knocking seven shades of shit out of each other before I know it.

1 March

Bronagh is saying 'dada'.

I'm not sure if this counts as her first word.

Colm is delighted.

At the moment, if Colm is 'dada' to Bronagh, then I'm the other sound she makes, which is a prolonged fart noise. Pretty accurate.

6 March

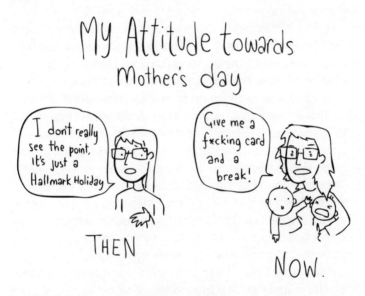

My Attitude towards Mother's day

I don't really see the point, it's just a Hallmark Holiday

THEN

Give me a f*cking card and a break!

NOW.

I love my kids. I love them more than I've loved anyone and that's scary. I worry a lot that I'm not a good enough mum, that I'm not attentive enough or I'm selfish. Or that because sometimes babies aren't easy company then that's bad. Or because I'm not this person saying, 'Motherhood is the most amazing thing in the world.' I just want to do right by them; if life is an adventure then Colm and I are their guides for the start of it. And I want them to have a great adventure.

7 March

Boss-level parenting: looking after two seven-month-old babies when both parents have vomiting and diarrhoea.

It came on really quickly last night when I was waiting for Colm to come home from London. The babies had woken up crying, then it started for me and I had to leave the room to go to our bathroom at the other end of the house. I had horrific diarrhoea before making my way back to them, feeling weak. Then I carried them downstairs because I didn't know what was happening.

Then I had to leave them again because I needed the toilet for a second time. As I made my way back, having lost so many electrolytes so quickly, both my hands cramped open and I was unable to close them.

I had to talk to Colm on speaker as he was in a taxi from the airport and I wasn't able to hold the babies, who were crying. Up to that point it was one of the scariest things to have happened to me as a parent.

Colm came home.

I threw up in the sink, not making it to the bathroom, then followed through as I stood there.

That happened again. Having puked into the nappy bin, this time I threw up into a bucket while sitting on the toilet. Colm felt sick and weak too.

The whole time the babies – the carriers of disease – were there and needed attention.

Colm and I basically had to tag-team it. One of us did something then felt weak, then the other stepped in until the same thing happened and we swapped again. We made it through the night, and back at 8 p.m. when this all started, the night seemed really f**king long.

This morning I had hiccups beside the babies. My hiccups are incredibly loud and the girls found them hilarious.

Babies, eh?

My friend Shaun took the girls to the crèche as Colm

and I were too weak and sick to do it.

He is my hero.

Colm and I spent the day in bed drinking MiWadi and Dioralyte. Colm puked into an empty biscuit tin.

At 5 p.m., both still feeling weak and nauseous, we mustered enough energy to collect the girls from crèche.

The first thing we see when we leave the house?

A seafood delivery van.

9 March

The babies are now perfect cuddling size. I told Colm, 'They're the size of a decent fairground prize.'

The downside of this is I can't carry them both at the same time any more. They're too big and too wriggly. When I'm carrying Róisín and she's facing forwards, she sort of pedals in the air, mostly when she sees something that excites her. I've started using her as a detector to find anything with which she might like to play – the more she pedals the more attractive the thing we are near to is. Unfortunately, Bronagh seems to be a less enticing prospect than the cat, who Róisín views as this mysterious fuzzy thing that appears sometimes and she knows to be soft (she's petted her a few times).

On the other hand, the cat views the babies as the things occupying mine and Colm's laps (which are rightfully hers) and Bronagh is more excited by Róisín than by the cat. So much so that she has a special squeal which means, 'Look, it's Róisín!'

And Róisín has a special squeal which means, 'Look, it's the cat!'

13 March

A lot of Colm's friends have kids – but he's two years older than me – and a lot of my friends don't have kids as they're younger than me. I can appreciate why people don't want kids, but right now I can't imagine life without mine in it.

I feel a lot of intense love for them, which is so powerful it makes me wonder why everyone doesn't want to feel like I do. However, telling someone they should have kids because you get a kick out of having kids is like pushing a drug. You might feel amazing being a parent, but all that your friends without kids see is you looking wrecked and having no money.

There's a common misconception that having kids universally binds people: 'You have kids? Well, you're part of our gang now!' People with kids don't all necessarily get on, though. The majority of my conversations with other parents in playgrounds or in crèche can be summed up by this Venn diagram:

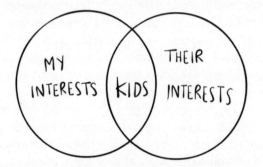

Also, I find myself only able to identify parents through their children. I don't know their first names – I just know them as [insert child's name]'s mum/dad.

Sometimes it feels as if having kids can be a divider, that I'm treated differently now I'm a mother, and that sometimes 'having kids' and 'having cancer' are said in the same hushed tones. As if I've been condemned to some terrible fate that you wouldn't want to think about or deal with.

I get that. But it is a choice. I wanted to do this – to invite this change into my life – but fundamentally I am still the same person. Being a parent isn't contagious. You can't 'catch the babies' off someone: 'I was around Ann – she has kids – and then, after I left, three babies fell out of my fanny so now I HAVE KIDS!'

Sometimes I do feel as awkward around friends who don't have children as they feel around me. Introducing people to babies is challenging too, because it's not like introducing them to a new boyfriend of yours. They're unlikely to have a lot in common and I'm not allowed to break up with the babies. Typically, introducing a baby to someone new, who doesn't usually like kids, goes like this:

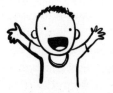

MOST OF THE DAY

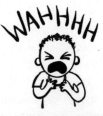

WHEN INTRODUCING THEM TO A FRIEND.

Being a parent can be lonely – the lack of free time, the inability to go out whenever you like, or even being unable to 'go for a drink after work' can all be isolating. Knowing that having kids has made me some sort of social leper doesn't help this either. I'm sure things will figure themselves out but it's hard. I want people in my life who understand what having kids is like, I want people who don't but will at least laugh at me when I talk about them, and I want people who don't have kids because sometimes you get tired of talking about kids all the time.

Kids.

15 March

We woke up at 7 a.m. on a Sunday.

Which is ridiculous.

I think we were the only ones awake.

Us, the guy on the radio, and people too excited about mass to sleep.

By 10 a.m. we were in the Botanic Gardens, having already eaten breakfast. For the babies, breakfast means 'eating porridge while repeatedly dropping on the floor the piece of banana mum gave us.'

This is what babies do to you.

Get you up early.

Get you out of the house.

Get you using the phrase, 'Sure, the day's half over!'

Now, when we take the babies places, often they want to have a look about. Róisín was asleep in the Botanic Gardens so I picked up Bronagh and held her outwards so she could look around. Also, so I could pretend she was Kuato from *Total Recall*.

There was this fountain she really liked; it was her first time seeing one. It's a pretty crap fountain, so it's a good starting point. Imagine if I'd shown her a really great fountain and then this poor one – she'd think all fountains were like the first.

Or love them all equally.

While Róisín was still asleep, we thought Bronagh might want to experience what grass feels like underfoot. She loved it. She scrunched it up in her toes, shouted at it, and drooled like crazy because that's what they do these days when they're concentrating or excited. It was pretty cool.

A wee while later I felt bad that Róisín had slept through it all. We put Bronagh back in the buggy and took out Róisín, who had just woken up and seemed really dazed.

I let her feel the grass with her feet.

No reaction, slight confusion.

I rubbed her feet over and back on the grass.

She wasn't into it and it just started to look like I was trying to clean dog poo off her.

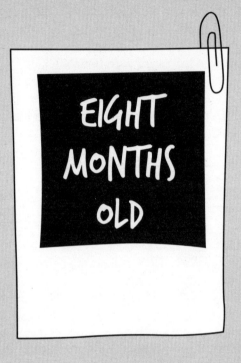

16 MARCH – 15 APRIL

* Says 'mama' and 'dada' to both parents (not specific)

* Stands with support or while holding on to something

* Crawls

* Points at objects

* Turns away when finished eating

18 March

I was telling Colm, 'I'm reading a thread on the Irish Multiple Births forum about things to get for when the babies start wandering around!'

'Fly paper!' he replied. 'Lots of it!'

19 March

Some days I feel as if I'm going to be tired for ever.

A feeling not helped by Róisín being awake most of the night. Awake, awake and going 'ngggghh' every five seconds.

Basically, her way of saying, 'I'm awake, I'm not happy about it but I'm not quite upset – but seriously, no one else is allowed to sleep.'

Tired. For. Ever.

20 March

A local coffee shop popular with parents asks me to draw on one of their blackboards. I create this, they give me coffee.

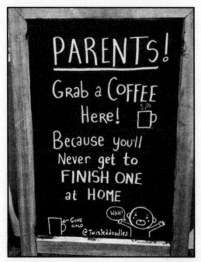

21 March

Last night Bronagh woke up at 3 a.m. She drank some of her bottle but was upset. I changed her nappy, which was wet, but she was still unhappy. Colm and I put her in our bed but she wouldn't settle, so we put her back in her cot and she got more upset – angry crying.

It was 4 a.m. by this point.

I told Colm there couldn't be anything else wrong with her, that she probably wanted to get back into our bed again. Now her crying was waking Róisín, who then got a nappy change and a bottle too.

Finally, Colm turns on the light, picks her up and brings her over to show her Róisín. She squeals happily at Róisín, Colm puts her back in her cot, she goes to sleep.

For whatever reason, Bronagh wanted to see that Róisín was OK.

Now that's been added to the list of 'possible reasons the baby is upset'.

Colm wins last night's parenting award.

Walking the babies home from crèche in their buggy, we stopped at some traffic lights. I shuffled the buggy over to make room for an old man with a walking stick to stand beside us.

He looked in the buggy, asked if they were twins.

Then he said to them, 'Well, ladies, may you always be as happy as you are right now.'

It made me want to cry.

25 March

I went to the cinema on my own today, then spent the rest of the time buying clothes for the babies as they are going up a size.

I told the cashier in Next that I had twins and was having a day to myself and that it was very exciting, that I had already been to the cinema by myself and had had ice cream. I told her I still feel compelled to look after them even when I'm not with them, hence the clothes-buying, but still it was exciting.

I asked if she had kids, she said no, but the cashier beside her said, 'I completely understand.'

'It's like day release from prison!' I said.

'Exactly,' she said.

'Except you probably have more sex in prison.'

'...'

Look at me making friends!

28 March

For a while, Bronagh has been using consonants in her speech. This is a thing: for ages, babies just cry, then they coo – which is mostly vowels. After that, there's the fart-noises stage and then it's babbling. Babbling is using consonants; it's where the whole 'dada' and 'mama' thing comes in. So developmentally, there has been a delay of maybe a week or so between the babies. Bronagh will do things first – such as smile, hence the Fun Baby/Dry Baby thing – so she was babbling while Róisín was still on fart noises. Then, when Róisín started babbling, it was great – I cried a little. Her voice is also different to Bronagh's – softer, more girly. Except now they both have colds and to be frank, Róisín sounds like the wee fella saying 'redrum' in *The Shining*.

Redrum.

Redrum.

Redrum.

29 March

The clothes for babies are amazing. I find myself standing in shops, holding sleepsuits which are adorable, and wanting to put my kids in them but also maybe wanting to wear them myself.

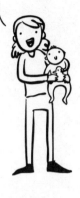

Baby clothes are so cute, I wish they made them in adult sizes.

DREAM

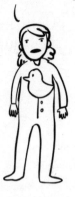

I look RIDICULOUS!!

REALITY

I've resisted dressing the babies the same. I'm aware of the idea that twins should be dressed in matching outfits but I don't know who that's for. I don't think it's for them, because they just want to be warm; I think maybe it's to enhance their 'twinness'. I want them to be individuals, though, so that means dressing them differently – or at least trying to.

They each have a colour scheme, more or less, which makes them sound as if they're rooms in a house. My friend Sarah dresses one of her kids in stripes and the other not in stripes. Essentially, you end up creating a 'home' and 'away' kit for your kids. Unfortunately, if you dress one kid in pink and the other in any other colour, the other child is assumed to be a boy.

HOW CLOTHING COLOUR HAS INFLUENCED STRANGERS WHEN GUESSING THEIR SEX.

PINK

girl!

BLUE

boy!

ORANGE

boy?

YELLOW

boy?

RED

boy!

GREEN

boy!

NAVY

boy!

PURPLE

girl? no wait, boy

WHITE

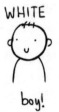

boy!

BLACK

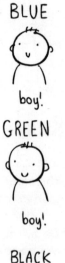

tiny Steve Jobs!

What? Boy? Is that a pipe?

Is that baby wearing mascara?

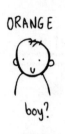
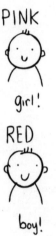

30 March

I get asked if I have a favourite baby.

My answer changes daily.

Some days it's hard to choose.

Some days there are no favourites.

Then, some days, one of the babies wakes everyone at 3 a.m. and stays awake for two hours.

Then it's fairly easy to choose.

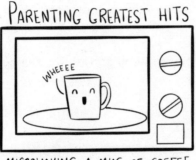

PARENTING GREATEST HITS

WHEEEE

MICROWAVING A MUG OF COFFEE

31 March

Colm came into the kitchen and told me, 'Bronagh is in her cot saying, "Mam mama mam mam mama."'

'Aw, is she talking about me?'

[*Awkward face*] 'I think she's trash talking you!'

Damn kids.

2 April

Some animals pretend to be dead to avoid being eaten by predators; some people pretend to be asleep to avoid parenting.

'The baby was crying really loudly? I didn't hear a thing!'

Noises that don't wake the babies up at night:

1. The TV
2. Traffic
3. The emergency services going past, sirens blaring
4. Students being drunk and shouting outside

Noises that wake the babies:

1. Colm and I making a cup of tea
2. Just making a damn cup of tea

Every night.

By the way, we aren't stirring the tea by blasting it with air horns.

3 April

The babies have discovered clapping. Bronagh likes to couple this newfound action with shouting. She looks like a tiny evangelical Christian.

Clapping doesn't seem like a big deal but, considering the idea that their hands could be brought together never even occurred to them for months, in baby terms it is a big deal.

The babies were sitting in Bronagh's cot today – they take turns to sit in each other's – and Róisín was clapping her hands. By the way, when I say clapping, they just bring their hands together, fingers spread. There is no noise, just a lot of action – like a mime orgy. So I clapped my hands in the same ridiculous style, fingers spread, while saying, 'YAY.' Róisín looked at me doing it, then she did it looking at me. Then I did it again, then we both did it, then Bronagh joined in.

On the surface we were all just idiots clapping our hands, me shouting 'yay' and making the most noise, but it was communication by imitation. They realized that they could copy me and, in turn, I was copying them.

I felt like the guy with the keyboard in *Close Encounters of the Third Kind*. This would make the twins the super-intelligent beings, although I don't think 'poking yourself in the eye with something you meant to put in your mouth' qualifies that notion.

Clapping isn't the only thing the babies have discovered recently. The worst thing they've discovered is jealousy. The emotion of war and *Jerry Springer*, of begrudgery and catty remarks, of crimes of passion and feelings of discontent.

That whole thing where people said to me, 'You'll have to buy two of everything!' Turns out, that doesn't matter.

Because even if you give them two of the exact same object, if one baby seems to be having more fun with it, the other will drop the object she's holding and take the other one. Playtime has basically become Grabfest/Keep Away. This was fine when they were just grabbing and dropping things. I would give the object back, and it was done in relative silence. That was fine – actually, it was even amusing. The winner of the Grabfest would generally shout and wave the object over their head in victory, then try to eat it. At which point it would be snatched back.

Shit got real this morning.

Róisín has discovered that if Bronagh takes something off her and she cries, Bronagh will not give it back.

But Colm or I will.

This has led to Bronagh grabbing the empty plastic bottle/spoon/[insert name of toy of which there are two but the kids have become fixated on one], Róisín crying while looking at us pointedly, and us giving the item back.

Bronagh has learned this trick too.

It. Is. The. Worst.

If I could undo one thing they've learned this weekend it would be this. This and the knowledge that it is now going to keep going until they're eighteen – and beyond.

Except later there will be words.

But also whingeing.

Whingeing with words.

'Muuuuummmm, Róisín stole my boyfriend/Nobel Prize/presidency...'

As an interesting aside, here are some of the things they have fought over: a tissue box, two rattles that are exactly the same, two wooden spoons that are exactly the same, Bronagh getting lifted out of the buggy first in the supermarket, toast, my phone which was turned off (this almost caused a riot – they don't know what's going on with my phone, why I like it but they want to find out), a silver hairbrush, a duck which makes a wibbling noise, and their feet.

From now on I'm going to be doing more peacekeeping than the UN, although I'm sure the UN's tactic isn't, 'If you can't play nicely neither of you gets this.' At which point they'd remove weapons/food/the Gaza Strip.

9 April

The babies have their own secret language. It's finally started.

They are super into each other but in a weird way. They can be side by side for ages, but if you hold one and the other looks at her, they have this moment of 'Oh my god, it's you!' Followed by an exchange of really excited squeals.

I've tried to join in with them by imitating the sounds that they make at each other. This has been met with more squealing.

We could be inciting genocide for all I know.

It's cute, though, but as with all cute things that babies do, they are cutest when done at a reasonable hour and when I'm not bolloxed tired.

11 April

Colm and I talk to a mortgage broker while the girls are at crèche.

The last few months, trying to get our finances in shape, have been trying. We have to buy a house – the rental market has imploded and looking at rental listings every night hasn't thrown up anything suitable or obtainable.

Colm is pushing this forward. I felt resistance – to the long-term commitment of putting down roots or saying, 'This is where we live now.' Our parents have given us some money towards a deposit. Colm's parents sold their home in Finglas and moved to Carlow, leaving the city so we can stay, and we are so grateful. My mum and dad helped out too. This feels like putting all our chips down on the table and hoping we can borrow enough. I don't know how this conversation with the broker would have gone if I'd given up my job – I'm glad I didn't. The broker gives us a figure for how much we can afford to spend on a house and suddenly we realize how few properties are within our budget.

WEANING

The babies are being weaned, and I don't know when this process stops. I feel like I'll be saying they're weaning for ever, but maybe they're done when they no longer drink bottles or when they move out.

Anyways, at this stage the babies are getting most of their food intake from 'not milk', which sort of suggests they're weaned?

Weaning is one of those 'choice areas' of parenting, where parents opt either for baby-led weaning or traditional weaning then judge parents who have chosen the other route. As far as I can tell, baby-led weaning

 continued...

involves putting food in front of the baby – usually something they can hold in their tiny idiot hands – and then letting them try to guide it to their ever-curious mouths.

Traditional weaning involves going crazy with a blender and spooning a variety of foods that seem to be either shades of white or orange into their ever-curious mouths.

Because Colm and I like to mock both sides of the parenting argument we are doing a combination of both approaches.

Letting the babies feed themselves sounds like a great idea. In fact, it involves me putting down more floor covering than Patrick Bateman after a house party, and having fleeting thoughts that the only thing that will thoroughly clean the high chairs after the babies are finished with their 'meal' is fire. Letting the babies feed themselves also involves me watching them like a hawk because I'm worried that baby-led weaning will turn into baby-led choking, and there's only so much hacking I can take before I give up and just f**k everything into the blender again.

That said, I worry that the main reason I like traditional weaning more, and seem to favour it, isn't that I enjoy the bond created by staring into my babies' eyes as I help them explore a world of flavours. It's more that I enjoy destroying food with our hand blender. I'd never used the hand blender before the babies came along but I have since used it to decimate a variety of meals that I have lovingly prepared.

The babies only eat with Colm and I at the weekends. During the week they are fed a variety of options (which sometimes contain the word 'casserole' or 'mash') by the crèche. I know this from the forms we get home at the end of each day, something which could be lied about except for one simple fact: the onset of weaning has led to a change in the babies' bowel movements.

continued...

I'd love to say it's been for the better, but the truth is, in the beginning, after a baby has cleared the black stuff (which looks like pure evil out of their bowel), their poops are shades of green or mustard-coloured and they don't really smell. You're changing nappies and thinking, 'Yes, this is OK. It's yellow, it smells vaguely of cheese. This isn't so bad, I can do this, I can deal with baby poo.' Then, over time, they get smellier, until you get into weaning and you're afraid to admit it, to admit the new truth that you are now cleaning proper adult poos off these finger-food-eating feckers. So yeah, the crèche says, 'We fed them beef casserole', and the next day that's 'beef asserole'. That's how I know they aren't lying.

The crèche doesn't really give the babies fish – well, not yet. To try to stop them being fussy eaters, I'm all for giving them fish. So this weekend they got salmon. To push the boat out I thought I'd give them salmon, avocado (the baby-weaning superfood/stain) and noodles. Yes, I made them cold soba noodles, put them into dashi (a broth) and served them with seaweed.

I am aware of how much of an asshole this makes me sound.

I felt like more of an asshole when I put the noodles – the cold, grey-brown noodles flecked with seaweed – on the high chair tables in front of the babies.

'What the f**k is this?' was written all over Róisín's face.

She went to touch them, then quickly withdrew her hand.

She looked at me. 'Is this some kind of a joke?'

In my mind, I thought the noodles would be fun for them, they could play with them and it would be nice, but no.

No. No. No. No. No.

The way the noodles looked tapped into something in their brain that said, 'This is not food, definitely not food,

continued...

I think it's worms, I don't know what they are but no.'
Apparently, some innate responses are hardwired into
our genetic code, such as how we know what snakes are,
but 'don't eat your own poop' has to be learned.

I thought it was interesting.

That said, our genetics obviously say nothing about
not eating the remote control or, I dunno, washing-
machine tablets.

I ate the noodles.

Then I destroyed a microwaved sweet potato with
the hand blender.

WEANING fashion for Mums!

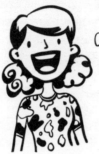

CLOTHES WITH
SPLODGES OF...

WHITE
ORANGE
AND GREEN

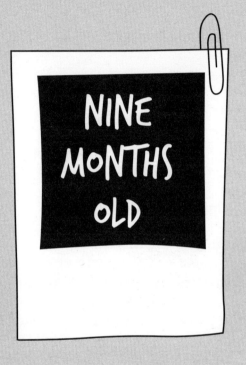

16 APRIL – 15 MAY

* Begins 'cruising' along furniture

* Drinks from a sippy cup

* Begins to eat with fingers

* Begins to bang objects together

* Displays separation and stranger anxiety

* Combines syllables into word-like sounds

17 April

The babies are growing at an alarming rate. It was inevitable; all that food had to be going somewhere. As I see them every day I don't really notice it – the growing – not until I'm scrolling through photos of them, on my phone, late at night. A reminder that time is moving on. Looking at pictures of them, in the dark, makes me miss them even though they are literally a light switch away. This is probably because babies use the act of sleeping to give the illusion that they aren't hard work.

For me, the more empirical measure that they're getting bigger is their clothing. They're now nine months old and in the back of my mind I am thinking about the next size up, 9–12 months, which seems to be a blind spot when we buy clothes as gifts.

Earlier today I stood in the spare bedroom, sorting clothes – some new, some second hand – into different sizes. An absolutely thankless task as the babies don't care what they're wearing as long as it's warm and they haven't pissed on it yet. These days I seem to spend more time dealing with clothes than I would like. Babies seem to go through more outfit changes than Beyoncé in concert, and then there are my clothes and Colm's too.

I'm trying to be more organized. I sort out socks and underpants, I fold Colm's clothes and put them away. I open the wardrobe door and throw my stuff on top of the cloth orgy that is my part of the wardrobe. I don't have the heart to sort out my things yet. I still don't fit into some of the less forgiving items and am having a Mexican stand-off with my body: it refuses to fit into my old clothes and I refuse to buy new ones to accommodate my new form.

It rained this morning. It was a lovely day and then it rained. I had clothes on the washing line. They are now wet, but they were probably almost dry. This is something I find myself getting annoyed about as I'm sorting out the clothes, but then I can't find a second pair of baby trousers that have pictures of cats on their knees so I get annoyed about that instead.

As I stand here, I remind myself of my own mother.

Her battle with laundry seemed endless. Incoming rainclouds heralded a cry to 'get the clothes in off the line' and out we ran into falling raindrops, clothes pegs clattering to the ground as each item was yanked down to safety.

My mother always seemed to be sorting out laundry. Washing it, drying it and spending countless hours ironing. I rarely iron, unless the item of clothing in question needs to look smart rather than slept-in. Even then I will definitely try to trick Colm into doing it for me.

As a kid, I think I assumed that my mother enjoyed doing laundry. Because as a kid, I had to do what my parents told me, which meant that they could do what they wanted. And if they could do what they wanted, surely they would only do things that they enjoyed. So, by that logic, my mother must have enjoyed doing laundry.

I do not enjoy doing laundry.

I believe I should tell my kids this – just to make it clear that it is not something I enjoy and that they should do their best not to dirty their clothing.

But they will probably forget I told them.

Just as I assume I've forgotten that my mother once told me.

And I'll have to wait for them to have kids of their own before they can appreciate this endless, thankless chore.

But...

Seriously, those clothes were almost dry.

PARENTHOOD IS BASICALLY STARTING A TINY ODD SOCK COLLECTION

I guess it's time I sorted out the laundry.

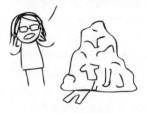

Don't get shirty with me, shirty.

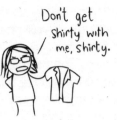

Pull yourself together, curtains!

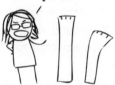

No flies on you, tiny baby Jeans.

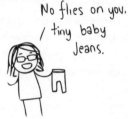

Don't get yourselves into a twist, knickers.

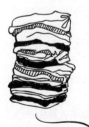

Are you Just saying Puns?

Yes! Because this job is stupidly boring

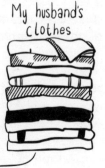

The babies' clothes

My husband's clothes

Mine

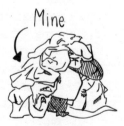

folded nicely

Flung into Wardrobe

23 April

WE ARE ON HOLIDAYS! I haven't left Dublin in over a year but now we're in Galway. We brought both of our nine-month-olds on the train to get here and it feels as if we've had to bring fifty bags of stuff. They loved the train, the people on the train loved them, and they loved the people on the train.

I can't lie, I was massively anxious about this whole trip but here we are.

I'm realizing that going on holiday with kids is like going to work in a different office for a few days: same shit, different location. The babies will have their own room, though, so we won't have to tiptoe around them as they sleep, and when we get up we'll be able to see the sea.

My parents used to bring us to Galway on holiday as children, Colm's parents used to bring their family here as children, so we're bringing our children here. It makes me wonder where Galway parents take their children? Probably Tenerife.

30 April

Today I went to an emotional well-being workshop set up by the multiple births group. To be honest, I only went because another twin mum, Jackie, was going. We met at the antenatal class we both went to last year but, despite the fact that we live incredibly near to each other, we've never managed to meet up. That's what happens – or doesn't happen – when you're trying to plan something around four babies.

I thought that maybe the workshop would be a bit of arse and that I wouldn't get anything from it, but I did. For the first time since giving birth, I was in a room with other multiple mothers. Suddenly, having two babies wasn't something that set me apart, it was something that included me. Apparently, in the past there had been a triplet mother at some workshops, and one class had a triplet mother *and* one of quadruplets. I said that if I had quadruplets, I'd begin every sentence, 'Well, as a mother of quads...' and then hope nobody would think I'd given birth to four-wheel vehicles.

Although the fact that each of us was a mother of multiples was unifying, there were things that set us apart: our experiences around becoming parents, how we had got there – be it through IVF or naturally, being able to bring home babies immediately or having to spend time in the NICU – and how the journey had affected us.

Empathy works best if you've had a similar experience. I have twins and I don't feel like I can identify with singleton mothers. Not because of them, but because of me. I don't want to hear them tell me that they know what it must be like to have twins, or that they can imagine what it's like, or that they can't, or that I must have it really tough, or that they have it tougher.

I was one of a few women in the workshop who had been diagnosed with postnatal depression. What helped each of us differed, but we were able to put a name to it. There were some women there who were still inside it, experiencing it, afraid to name it. More than anything I hope that workshop helped those women to know that it's OK. Just because you have shit going on, it doesn't make you weak or less than anyone else. The desire to sort your shit out, that's what makes you stronger, but the hardest steps are getting to that point. Or something like that. I just hugged people and told some of them that I understood, because I did.

When I'm in a room of people who all have two babies, other factors come into play. As much as I am a twin mother, I have no idea what it is like to go through round after round of IVF, to lose those babies, to finally get two miracles and feel so frightened that you might lose them.

I also carried my babies 'full term' so I have no idea

what it is like to visit your little ones in a neonatal unit, be obsessed with them gaining weight, getting better, seeing them get worse, waiting for them to come home, bonding with them, and worrying in that way.

Empathy is a funny thing. We strive to connect and rework our own experiences in an attempt to angle them to someone else's point of view in their particular situation, but sometimes we fail. Sometimes the fear of failure is enough to make us not want to go there, or the fear of even having to put ourselves in that imaginary situation.

I do not know what it is like to have a very sick baby.

I do not want to know what it is like to have a sick baby.

I do not want my babies to get sick.

So I cannot go there.

And for all that I say, 'I cannot imagine how hard that is . . .' I want to hear their story.

One thing I have realized is that although other parents may not know what it's like to have two babies at the same time, there are certain things that unite us.

We love our kids.

We are all watching them grow and when it comes to that there are certain things that are almost universal . . .

We've all dealt with a full-body poo, where it goes up their backs and outside the nappy and it feels like it will never come off their skin.

We may not know how to relate to the figurative shit other parents have gone through but we're united by the literal shit.

3 May

The babies keep dropping their spoons on the floor. I keep picking them up. Apparently, this is how they test the way the world works – doing the same thing repeatedly to see if they get the same result. I have no idea who is funding this spoon study.

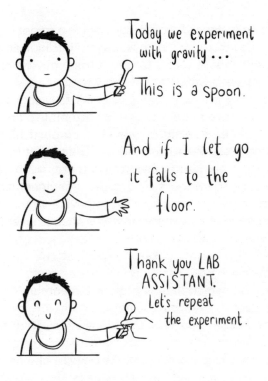

6 May

This week the babies have mostly been teething.

Teething is one of those things which explain why your baby is crying.

In the beginning it's usually wind, then it's colic and then it's teething.

'Why won't the baby stop crying?'

'She is unsheathing her fangs.'

For a while the babies had two teeth each. The lower central incisors are meant to come up first, then the upper central incisors. Then, after that, the upper lateral incisors, which are the teeth either side of the central ones.

The mouth, it seems, is a place of order. In truth, there is very little a baby can do with two teeth on its lower jaw – other than open beer bottles, possibly.

To be awkward, Róisín has decided to get her lateral upper incisors first, which is making her look like a small vampire. I would take a photo of them but it's hard to get her to open her mouth and show them, and every time I take out my phone these days she lunges at it.

It's not even as if we give her the phone when it's on and show her amazing things on it. I hand it to her with the screen blank and she drools manically, turning it over and over in her hands, trying to discover its mysterious secrets before biting it repeatedly with her vampire uppers.

Bronagh is also getting two teeth, but a central incisor and a lateral incisor – two teeth joining the party in her mouth without their partners. I think this means that they will both get all four of these teeth in quick succession, which means prolonged teething.

Teething is, of course, teeth coming into play, but it's also accompanied by the following symptoms: red cheeks, runny noses, low-grade fever, lack of appetite, horrendous poos, and generally being a cranky arse.

Runny noses can cause postnasal drip, which can lead to a cough, and coughing at night can result in a baby becoming a babbling milk fountain. A milk fountain that isn't happy that it's been sick, needs to be changed – along with the bed – and isn't allowed more milk.

Late nights and difficulties aside, it's weird to watch teeth appear – the babies are becoming small people. It's a bit like putting a face on Mr Potato Head – before, he's just a potato.

8 May

Colm and I have been looking at different houses, including the one we're in, in terms of what we are going to buy. The house we are in has character – in that we have to hold open the windows with books; the bathroom is at the furthest part of the house, past the kitchen; and the floor in the sitting room is at such an angle that if the girls roll a ball away from them, it will come back. However, it has been our home for almost two years. It is the place we brought our babies back to when they were born. We love it and we know it. It might be too much of a task to take on, though, as it needs a lot of renovation. The landlord wants to sell it but he has said he will show it with us still in the house, which is accommodating of him, but I hate living in this limbo. I want a home.

10 May

Today the public health nurse saw Bronagh, naked and screaming, empty her bladder on to a changing mat, pissing from an assisted standing position on to the plastic below her. The public health nurse isn't very good at comforting upset babies, probably because she runs her clinic like Guantanamo Bay.

'Strip her down. I want to weigh her.'

From the start, Bronagh was not a fan of this approach. She didn't like the woman. She doesn't like strangers telling her to smile either, telling her to smile and then stripping her down.

I'm wiping piss off the mat using tissue, the nurse isn't really comforting Bronagh, and Róisín is looking on from the buggy. She must be vaguely amused because she's not crying. She has no idea what's going on.

Bronagh is sitting on the weighing scales and crying, but I can't touch her or comfort her. Once I'm allowed to dress her – something else she isn't happy about – the nurse persists in asking me questions and the sweat is rolling off me. Bronagh is still crying and all I want to say to the nurse is, 'Shut up for a minute until I comfort her.' But I answer the questions, and we sit beside the nurse.

She offers Bronagh a pen. Bronagh cries – she doesn't want a pen, not from this woman. I give her my keys instead, then my phone, which is turned off, but she starts shouting at it, delighted. The keys *and* the phone – surely this is a special day.

The nurse asks more questions.

'Is she pointing yet?'

I am unsure. Bronagh knows what to do when she sees something she wants. She waves and reaches for it and shouts, but she's not exactly choosing sofas out of the IKEA catalogue.

'Yes,' I answer.

'Does she sit unassisted?'

'Unassisted, yes. Trusted and unassisted? No.'

Is she sitting up on her own? Is she trying to pull herself up? Does she say things? Can she use the pincer grasp? Does she make strange?*

I have no idea why she even asked that last question considering what had happened.

Róisín took it all in her stride, smiling throughout. The nurse praised her, saying how great she was. Yes, because she wasn't losing her shit at some stranger messing with her.

It was easier this time, but back in the buggy Bronagh wasn't happy and wanted to leave.

First, we had to finish the same process of weighing, answering questions, checking Róisín's length.

'Will you dress them the same?'

'No. They're two different people.'

The nurse asks how I am, how I'm coping, but not with any concern, more with the bored voice of someone who has boxes to tick and wants to tell me stories about babies drinking bleach and electrocuting

---

* Meaning to act up, be nervous or shy in the presence of a stranger, or when in a strange situation. The phrase seems to be loaned from Irish – *'coimhthíos a dhéanamh le duine'* literally means 'to make strangeness with someone', or to be shy or aloof in their presence – but there are similar phrases in Finnish, German, Portuguese and Spanish.

themselves. I don't tell her about the postnatal depression.

I realize that I'm glad I have someone else to talk to about that, because this woman wouldn't get it. She's in a room with someone trying to deal with two babies at the same time and she's about as useful as a foam finger in a delivery suite.

I take a note of the babies' lengths and weights. She tells me the lengths aren't accurate, and I wonder why she took them. What was the point?

Bronagh is still bigger, but not by a huge margin. Both babies are longer than average and lighter than average. Later, Colm says, 'They get that from me.'

'Thanks for making me feel fat,' I grumble.

Even though the nurse said, 'You're wasting away', which I didn't take as a compliment.

Today Colm and I have been married for three years, and the emotion of that comes and goes in waves, bringing me to near tearful moments. The crèche did a picture with the girls, using their handprints. It says 'Happy Anniversary' and it makes me cry.

Whenever I think back to our wedding my memories of it get fonder and fonder. At the time, there wasn't anything I would have changed about the day and I stick by that. Earlier this evening, when I'm home with the babies and playing music, the song 'Can't Hold Us' by Macklemore and Ryan Lewis comes on the radio and I dance to it with the babies in turn.

That song reminds me of the day I got married.

Not that it was played at the ceremony. I think it was played later – during the disco – but I'd listened to it as I walked into town on my own that morning to get my hair and make-up done because I was going to get married.

Colm and I were going to get married in a zoo and nothing was going to f**k that up.

And nothing did.

I don't often say these things, but I consider myself

incredibly lucky. For the people I know, the people who love me, those who have been in my life at the right moment, and even at the wrong moment.

I have a husband who is my best friend, has excellent parenting skills and contributed top-class genetic material to our kids, even if they do kick him in the balls occasionally.

Did I think when I got married that I would spend our third wedding anniversary wiping the piss of one of our identical twins off the changing mat belonging to the public health nurse?

No, bloody hell, no, but how brilliant is that?

GHOST OF PARENTING FUTURE

At some point, my interactions with strangers about the babies have shifted from 'Aren't they very small and lovely?' to 'Once they start crawling you . . . are . . . f**ked.'

I also get, 'Imagine how hard it's going to be when they are both toddlers.'

Usually the exchange ends with 'Enjoy them, the time passes so quickly.'

THANKS, STRANGERS!

If parenting was a movie being shown at the cinema, it would involve all the people who have already seen it, shouting spoilers at those waiting to go in – spoilers that give you the impression that those people f**king hated the movie – but then they finish with 'ENJOY THE MOVIE. IT'S GREAT AND IT IS OVER TOO SOON!'

I call these interactions 'ghosts of parenting future', where people feel the need to warn you about things that are ahead of you when, in essence, you're just hoping to make it to the end of the day intact. The sort of people who, when you ask if it gets any easier, reply, 'It doesn't get easier, it's just different.'

continued...

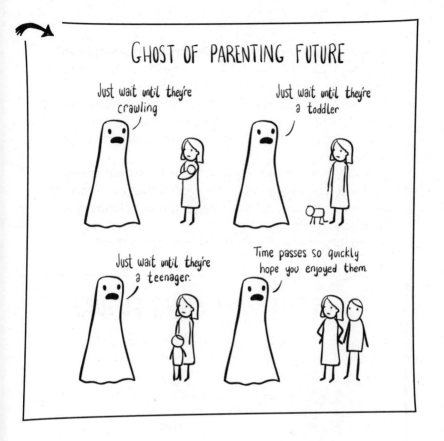

UNSOLICITED PARENTING ADVICE

Another interaction you have as a parent is when people try to give you advice on how to raise your baby, advice you didn't ask them for. One of the reasons for this is that most parents aren't 100 per cent confident in what they are doing, and the best way to give the impression that they do is by giving their opinion. It's like someone telling you how to complete a level on a computer game that they've just finished, even though their avatar was entirely different and there's every chance you're playing on another difficulty setting.

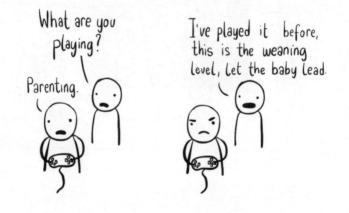

Although people's intentions are generally good when dispensing parenting advice, it can feel a bit much when you haven't asked for it.

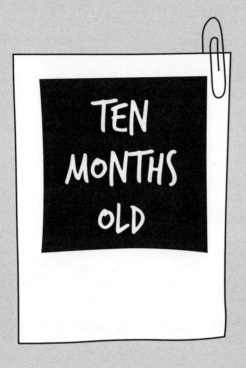

16 MAY – 15 JUNE

* Waves goodbye

* Eats well with fingers

* Picks up objects using pincer grasp

* Begins to understand the word 'no'

* Says 'mama' and 'dada' to the correct parent

16 May

'How do you tell your twins apart?'

'Well, one of them has ripped off her bib, is completely covered in food and has Weetabix from yesterday rubbed in her hair. The other hasn't.'

Top tip: Weetabix and milk make a great alternative to hair gel if you want to keep that my-sister-keeps-slapping-my-head look fresh all day.

17 May

Colm has passed his driving test! Hooray!

He is now getting car seats for the kids to drive them around in our car.

I've never even been in our car!

18 May

Someone stops me to talk about the twins.

'Girl and a boy, is it?'

'No, two girls.'

'Ah, you'll have to go again for a boy.'

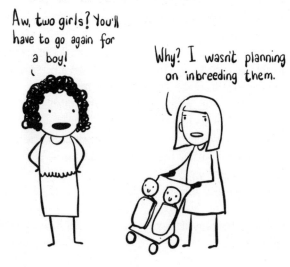

Aw, two girls? You'll have to go again for a boy!

Why? I wasn't planning on inbreeding them.

19 May

Colm has gone to London today so I did the whole dropping the babies (not literally) at crèche.

Róisín spent most of the morning crying while we were getting ready, which only stopped when I held her or if she saw some object she liked. If I left the room, she cried. Who am I kidding – she was crying before I even left the room. Bronagh now joins in. When I'm on my own I have to leave them to cry in a safe place while I get ready for work. This doesn't take long.

As I return they are crying.

They do not want yogurt with strawberries; they do not want water or milk. So I put them in the buggy.

They stop crying.

I take them to crèche and explain to the staff that Róisín has been having a bad morning.

But she's fine now. I mean, she's no longer crying.

Horrible thought: 'Róisín couldn't wait to get to crèche.'

A baby boy waddles across the room (he can walk, what a show-off) and Róisín is delighted. She stares at him. He's got that kind of gormless-looking face you see plastered on babies 95 per cent of the time. I know he can smile – I've seen him – so I smile at him. Nothing.

Bronagh stares at me, wondering if I'm hanging around for a reason, then gets vaguely upset when I go to leave. Róisín doesn't even look at me.

I put the buggy away, then, when I'm outside, I look in the window to the baby room.

Róisín is in a high chair, still staring at the boy. She doesn't even notice me standing outside in the rain, watching glumly.

'At least she isn't crying,' I think. And suddenly I feel worse.

I need to play it cool – babies don't want some needy mum.

I'll show up to crèche with another baby. That'll teach her.

But it is a terrible, terrible idea.

23 May

My parents came down to Dublin today. They were going to give Colm and I the night off so we could go out for a meal. It was a big deal, but when they arrived I could tell by the look on my mum's face that something was wrong. My uncle, my father's youngest brother, has died – they only found out on the way down. We've had a cup of coffee together but now they have to head back.

Colm has had his driving licence for less than a week, has spent his entire time driving around Dublin and has now been lumped with the task of driving me and two ten-month-old babies, who have only been in a car twice before, on a four-hour trip to Donegal.

The trip does not take four hours, though, it takes six, as we have to stop the car to feed the babies and change them, to entertain them. Someone told me to have a bag of snacks, toys and soothers with me in the front seat so I can pass them back in rolling succession.

24 May

The funeral is huge and we carry the babies with us into the graveyard, where I meet so many of my relatives who I haven't seen in years. I introduce them to the babies and some of them to my husband, who they have never met before. It is an incredibly warm day, with the sun beating down.

We stay at my parents' but before we leave Donegal we take the babies to the beach I used to visit as a child. They marvel at the sand, squealing and crushing it in their small hands, before they start to eat it. They don't understand that sand isn't a food that someone has over-seasoned with salt or why we have to take them away from it.

The trip home takes seven hours. Towards their bedtime we change the babies into sleepsuits in a supermarket car park to prepare them for sleep and send them the message that yes, this is bedtime, but no, we are not home yet.

We do get home in one piece, though. I am so proud of Colm and his driving skills – he did so well.

25 May

I picked up the girls from crèche today, as I always do, bringing out their buggy from the buggy room that smells like feet. Dragging it into the hall and unfolding it is a bit like helping a drunken Transformer.

In the early days I tried to stick to a system where I wouldn't pick up the same baby first two days in a row. I figured they'd be keeping score, but my system has now collapsed into 'who is physically closest when I come in?'

It was Róisín today, as Bronagh had pooped herself and so was being changed. Then Bronagh came back and used her only means of communication – whining – to let me know that she would like me to hold her.

When it comes to putting them in the buggy, I settle Bronagh in and she whines so I give her her soother. I then go to pick up Róisín, who cries, but reaches for her crèche worker, who takes her. When she does, Róisín stops crying.

This. Is. New.

I am suddenly not the best and most amazing person that the babies know.

F**k.

And it feels like a punch in the gut.

Róisín chose someone else over me.

F**k.

I make a joke about it, telling the crèche worker maybe not to be so good at her job, to give Róisín a rough time tomorrow so I'm back on top. But I am still devastated.

I feel the need to win Róisín over later.

I think about what I could give her that would make me her favourite again. Ridiculous thoughts about treats and feelings of guilt wash over me.

People spoil their kids.

'They've spoiled their kids – they've given them too much,' I used to think. 'They get anything they want. That's a terrible way to raise a child. Why would you do that?'

I didn't understand it, not really. Not until now.

I think people spoil their kids for a number of reasons, one of them being so they feel like less of an asshole for leaving them in a crèche, with a childminder, or with a nanny while they go to work. They spoil their kids so that they will like them and so that their kids know they love them even though they can't give them all their time.

And Róisín wants to stay with the crèche worker.

And I feel like an asshole.

And I want to win her back.

But I don't want to spoil her to make myself feel better.

Colm comes back home. After a fight to get them to sleep, the babies are in bed finally. I tell him what happened at the crèche.

'That's pretty normal, I think. She was having fun there, you came to stop that, so she complained.'

'Does she hate me?'

'No.'

'Am I a bad mother?' I ask this in a whiney voice, crying, and now I know where Bronagh gets it from.

'No, you're a good mother.'

I now wonder if this is how babies work: they spend months letting you think that you're amazing, you're the best, all they want is Mammy, even Daddy isn't as good as Mammy.

It's flattering and surprising and you get used to it.

Then, your celebrity status gets eroded slowly by other people and by the babies being upset at you, because their world is expanding and your world is mostly them.

It is shit.

Like someone in a failing relationship, I have to resist the urge to spice things up, buy them toys – things they like – and remind them of the good times. Cue me showing them photos of us together while trying to avoid the ones where anyone looks upset.

But, I'm guessing this is normal.

I tell myself that.

Colm tells me that.

Google tells me that.

It is OK.

That evening, in an attempt to clear the babies' stubborn nappy rash, I give them a bath in salt water. This results in a frenzy as they love water. Eventually the two of them are in the bath, naked, splashing themselves, each other, the room and me.

They are happy.

I am happy but worried about how much they will cry when I take them out. They do cry. They want to go back in the bath. The bath was fun and I stopped it.

I am Mammy.

Wiper of tears and bums, and a fun sponge.

Later, I try to get Róisín to say 'Mammy', but all she wants to say is 'hiya' and wave at things.

She should be on a float in a parade.

28 May

Though the twins now sit on the floor mostly, or in their cots, there is still that blind there's-something-over-there-I-want-to-see-so-I-will-try-to-move-towards-it idea implanted.

They're idiots.

But getting less idiotic in different ways.

Suddenly, they're both doing the pincer grip. That's the grip where you pick things up using your thumb and forefinger, otherwise known as a 'normal grip', otherwise known as 'wait, there's another way to pick things up?'

Yes, there is.

Using your whole hand to grab something.

That is what has been happening until now.

They still grab at things – namely hot beverages I'm trying to drink while they are sat on my lap – but for smaller things they pull out the pincer grip.

Putting things in things. This is another milestone. Earlier today I was playing with Bronagh by putting a beer mat in my mouth (I realize how classy this is making me sound) and she would pull it out, then put it back in. At one point she dropped it and it went down my top. I fished it out, but she kept trying to put it back down my top.

Who's the classy one now?

This is her thing, you see. She likes dropping things and wants to know where they've gone – if they've disappeared – because before this, she believed that everything she couldn't see simply disappeared because the universe was created by her and to suit her.

She's still getting over it.

What a bloody let down, eh? You think you created the universe and even bloody beer mats won't obey your will.

Róisín, on the other hand, really likes to put things in her mouth. Such things include socks, leaves we hand her to examine, and bits of plastic she comes across on the floor that I realize she has found only when she starts gagging on them. Now I have to be hyper-alert for tiny bits of bloody plastic and choking hazards on the floor!

An interesting fact: sometimes they don't want to eat their food, possibly because cottage pie cannot compare to the gastronomic wonder of one of my socks; it simply doesn't have the same depths of flavour they are used to.

That said, they often want to eat *my* food. Today, we were eating out. I ordered something for myself and something for them. They didn't want their mashed potato with mashed carrot, but apparently my penne all'arrabiata was fine. So I end up giving them my food, all the while thinking, 'What is happening?! WHAT IS THIS?! THEY HAVE THEIR OWN FOOD BUT I CAN'T HELP MYSELF!'

30 May

This week I uttered the words 'our little babies are growing up', then made Colm sit with me and look at photos of them when they were born and a little older.

They *are* growing up but they're still babies – I can't send them down the shop for some milk, or even into the kitchen for some milk.

Or even ask if they know what the kitchen is.

Or milk.

Or...Oh, for feck's sake, where did you find that bit of plastic...?

BABY MAGIC

1. CHECK THE FLOOR

THERE'S NOTHING THERE!

2. PUT THE BABY ON THE FLOOR.

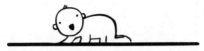

3. TA-DA! A BUTTON/COIN/CAT FOOD MAGICALLY APPEARS IN THEIR HAND.

1 June

Trying to buy a house is the worst. No wonder nobody ever got out of the car in Game of Life. They lived in that car and just piled it full of kids.

We've viewed, bid and been outbid on a number of houses now. It is heartbreaking. Whenever we go to a viewing, we often see the same people also looking for homes, and some of them are very nice. We make jokes but underneath is the fact we're all just looking for a home. Each time Colm and I decide, 'This house, I think we could make this work,' I can't help but imagine that it is our home. However, whenever we put in a bid someone else then talks to the estate agent and tells them they're willing to pay more. So you up your offer and the same phone calls happen again. All of these unseen people push us further into uncertainty, then the property in question goes to someone else and we find ourselves back to a house we can't stay in but can't leave, because we have nowhere to go.

8 June

It is incredibly warm today. Inflating a children's paddling pool in the hot sun, using a hand pump, is

What are you looking for in a Home?

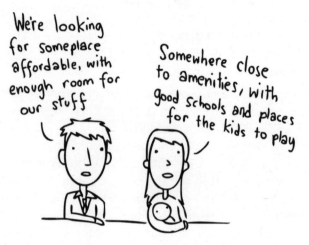

We're looking for someplace affordable, with enough room for our stuff

Somewhere close to amenities, with good schools and places for the kids to play

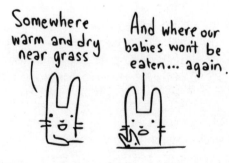

Somewhere warm and dry near grass

And where our babies won't be eaten... again.

surely one of the circles of hell. The thing had five different valves and I didn't have time to read the instructions. My children were hot and cranky, and although yesterday's set-up of one in the baby bath, one in a basin had gone OK, I felt bad for Bronagh being in a basin, which she was moving around the back yard simply by shifting her weight. This also meant the basin frequently had to be refilled.

We did try two in the baby bath but there is only so much of being kicked in the fanny by your sister that a baby can take.

The upside, despite the fact I had to sit in the hot sun playing lifeguard at a fish-shaped paddling pool?

They loved it.

9 June

Before I had babies, I had never read *The Very Hungry Caterpillar*.

I had no need to – I assumed it was just about a caterpillar that was hungry.

I've since read it and it is indeed about a caterpillar that is hungry.

In fact, the whole thing reads like someone doing pretty well on a diet during the week and then, come Friday, eats everything around him – cheese, sausages, cakes, pickles, salami.

On the Sunday he pulls it back and eats a single leaf.

Then comments about how fat he's become, hides himself away for two weeks, and comes back as a fabulous butterfly.

I am no stranger to this story, because the babies keep wanting me to read it. Today I read it four times because Róisín protested when it was over the first time and then smiled when I started it again. And because I like that they like me reading to them.

The babies are almost eleven months old and are

demonstrating that they have a will. Before this – well, in the early days – they were driven by hunger and seeking out comfort. Anything that interfered with those needs provoked a response: crying, always crying. I dealt with it, but then it was about liking certain foods, or if I showed them a toy they might show interest in it, but as soon as it was gone they'd forget about it. Then it would come back and they'd like it again.

Now, not only are they demonstrating that there are things that they like, but they also remember things. If I take them to the park, Róisín will get excited when she sees the swing – so excited that she starts to whine because I don't put her in it quickly enough.

Then she's happy enough.

It's a cliché but they really are becoming little people, with likes and dislikes. They could probably fill in some sort of 'baby date' profile now.

Likes: swings, *The Very Hungry Caterpillar*, bubbles, strawberries.

Dislikes: being taken out of the swing, teething, my sister getting more attention than me.

Because, oh yes, the jealousy thing is creeping in. They are starting to fight – it can even get a bit UFC at times, mostly hair-pulling but one did try to bite the other. They both want to sit on me, to be cuddled by me, to be played with at the same time. It can be a bit intense.

The crying, however, isn't proper crying. It's the whingeing of someone who is trying to exert their power of choice without having the vocabulary or physical ability to do it. Being a baby must suck.

I can read *The Very Hungry Caterpillar* whenever the hell I want.

I simply choose not to.

BABY BOOK IDEAS

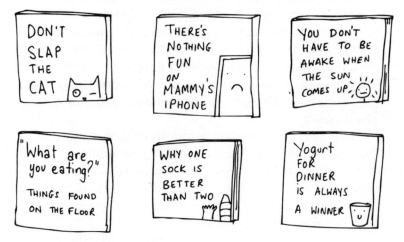

DON'T SLAP THE CAT

THERE'S NOTHING FUN ON MAMMY'S iPHONE

YOU DON'T HAVE TO BE AWAKE WHEN THE SUN COMES UP

"What are you eating?" THINGS FOUND ON THE FLOOR

WHY ONE SOCK IS BETTER THAN TWO

Yogurt FOR DINNER IS ALWAYS A WINNER

10 June

Good news: all of my hair that fell out a few months ago is growing back, so now it's all different lengths. It looks as if it was cut by someone pretending to know what layers are. Speaking of which, recently I tried to cut the girls' hair and it turns out I've no idea what I'm doing. Somehow it never occurred to me that they'd need a haircut at some point – I just assumed it would sort itself out. It doesn't. When my mother saw what I'd done to them she said, 'Well, at least it will grow out.'

WISPY TUFTS OF HAIR ARE SO IN RIGHT NOW

14 June

The baby monitor is acting up. Colm and I were watching TV this evening when this robotic baby cry came through the unit. So we did the only thing we could do...

We nicknamed them Robot and Brobot.

Also, there's nothing like googling 'weird noises baby monitor' and having horror movies come up in the search results.

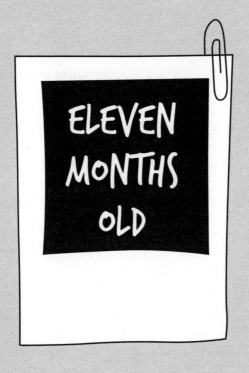

16 JUNE – 17 JULY

* Plays patty-cake and peek-a-boo

* Begins to imitate others

* Stands alone for a couple of seconds

* Cruises along furniture

* Claps hands

* Puts toys into containers

* Indicates wants with gestures rather than crying

* Understands simple instructions

IT TAKES A VILLAGE

Motherhood used to be different. That saying, 'It takes a village to raise a child,' was more literal when you think that people used to have children in communities where their mother lived down the road or the neighbour who also had babies could look after yours while you were running some errands.

These days the communities are online – small groups of parents all reaching out to one another because it's hard to do it all on your own – and, like a village, you begin to recognize people, if only by their profile picture or username. You know their kids and their names. I was part of a small closed Facebook group, and all of us had twins or triplets. There was a shared spirit of 'this is crazy, isn't it?' I became friends with two mothers of twins: Jackie, who I'd met at the antenatal class, and Sarah, someone who I had never met. Sarah was a friend of a friend and she lives in London. We were thrown together when our mutual friend said, 'You both have twins, I think you would get on,' and we did.

Another friend of mine said that when you're a parent, the friends you make are people who have a similar attitude to parenting as you do. The parents I became friends with were people who found humour in the day-to-day and used that humour to save themselves from it. And because parenting involves spending a lot of time alone with small infants who – depending on the day – aren't eating, sleeping or pooping, we would send messages to one another. Messages that didn't need to be replied to straight away, but the act of sharing your woes meant you knew that someone with a similar sense of humour and confusion about the whole thing was there with you, in the same boat.

continued...

And we kept one another going.
And we made one another laugh.

I liked to use humour to connect with other parents because I was finding it all hard. The group I was in knew how to laugh, how to reassure and how not to judge. Sometimes, by talking about a problem, you find out that you aren't alone. However, as with all aspects of parenting, to parent is to be judged, so it's a good idea to keep in mind that some of the people involved in discussions don't know you, they don't know your kids, and sometimes they're looking for an excuse to make themselves feel better as a parent by making you feel worse. That's not how you become a better parent, though.

This is one of the problems I posted in the early days:

> I've three week old identical twin girls.
> They've recently started crying more, the newest development is both of them crying at the same time, often this will go on for an hour or so at ridiculous hours of the morning. My question is this, how could I get them to harmonize their crying? Possibly in the style of Destiny's Child?
> At this stage I'm afraid I'll have to auto tune them.

Most parenting groups feature certain categories of posts:

The I'm-not-looking-for-medical-advice-but-what-is-this-rash?: Where a photo of a rash is uploaded and people – usually without any medical background – try to guess what it is.

The photo pile-on: Any occasion where people can post snaps of their kids. You will see loads of pictures of children, and when you know the people involved it's

continued...

actually nice to see them growing up. However, you are also secretly hopeful that photos of your children will get the most likes.

The martyr: A response to a comment which implies that the poster works hardest as a parent. For example, when replying to a thread about TV shows, they'll write, 'I don't know how you get time to watch TV.' This also implies that time spent doing things that aren't parenting must mean you are somehow neglecting your children.

The parenting competition: This kind of post doesn't usually appear on forums where people know one another, but the best example I saw was a Facebook post from a company asking 'How many hours a night does your baby sleep for?' All it took was one person to answer '11' for a load of people to say '11' or '12', as if it were some kind of contest. I think the question was meant to create a discussion; it actually created a monster.

The has-anyone-bought-this-baby-equipment/ toy-and-is-it-any-good?: Some very real reviews follow, some buyer's regret and a few people will post their own photo of said item, hoping to sell it second-hand.

Back when I was pregnant I would google any problematic symptoms only to be shown posts from women on parenting forums asking the same thing. I didn't want that, I wanted a medical professional's advice. Then, after the babies were born, I'd google different problems only to be shown answers from medical professionals. This time around I didn't want that, I wanted to hear from someone who had gone through the same thing themselves.

I ended up soliciting advice – actually asking for it rather than being given it uninvited – which was often brilliant and made me feel like part of a community. In turn, I tried to answer other parents' questions to the best of my ability, or at least tried to raise a smile. That

continued...

said, one of my favourite things on parenting sites is the 'parenting problem brag', which isn't really someone with a problem looking for advice. It is essentially a brag dressed up as a problem and there are bonus points for getting two brags into the same post:

> My two-year-old, who has been eating broccoli since he was twelve months, keeps complaining that his glasses won't stay in place while he's trying to read *Ulysses*. Am I being unreasonable in asking him to simply adjust the book's position?

What you need to know:

You are an amazing mother, you are doing a brilliant job and no one knows your children better than you.

You have nothing to feel guilty about.

That needs to be said and you need to believe it. I think that parenthood is about feeling guilty. Then, when your kids grow up, you bat the guilt back to them when you ask why they don't call any more.

21 June

Colm sends me yet another property listing. He's started looking beyond where we are living at the moment because it's becoming really obvious that we can't afford to live here. The house in question is blue, which I comment on straight away. It looks nice, but all the houses look nice. Then we go and have a look at the outside of it and the idea that we could live there is slowly crushing me.

He tells me about all the good things near the house – it's close to where he grew up. But the house isn't viewing any more so he's having to arrange for us to go and see it. I worry that this is a bad thing – the house is possibly haunted and no one wants it.

Types of Reply to a Problem on a Parenting Forum

Has similar problem which is actually reassuring.

Has similar problem but ten times worse like this is a "parenting woes" competition

Wants you to know that their child has never been any bother to them.

Had similar problem but solved it by simply being a better parent than you.

Has never had this problem and makes you feel like a bad parent or something is wrong with your kid

Impractical advice you initially laugh at but later try out of desperation.

Practical advice that worked for them. Every parent figures out their own way.

Someone saying "This problem is EASY, IT* GETS WORSE!!"

* BEING A PARENT.

22 June

'We're not keeping any baby clothes. This is it for us and babies. No more of them. No more clothes.'

This was my input into a conversation about storing baby clothes.

I am incredibly quick to point out that this is enough babies.

Two.

That's a good number.

Two.

I didn't see the point of keeping the clothes and our house is becoming overrun with bags of them. It's as if we are trying and failing to run a launderette.

'I'm keeping some of the clothes,' a co-worker told me, 'because some of the outfits are nice and they have good memories.'

I found this a bit ridiculous. Why would you keep baby clothes as mementos?

I am holding a baby dress, it has a pattern of lemons on it.

I am holding that small, lemony baby dress and I am crying.

The dress is sized 0–3 months, and there is also a strawberry dress, the sleepsuit with ducks, and the one with blue dots.

'They were so small,' I say out loud to no one, and snot escapes my nose.

As I am crying, I am trying to figure out why I am crying.

I miss my babies.

This is insane as they are literally in the next room.

I don't miss them, I miss them at the age they were when they were wearing these dresses. I miss those babies.

At the same time I am perfectly happy with the babies next door.

Babies change a lot.

Even if you knew someone who reinvented their look every week – say, Lady Gaga – she would never change as much as a baby does.

Or need to be changed as much as a baby does.

If at all. (She looks as if she's got a strong pelvic floor.)

Babies increase in size and weight at an alarming rate. If that happened to an adult, there would certainly be some sort of doctor's visit or intervention involved. In just a year, they go from these wrinkly, black-eyed blobs to looking like babies to looking like small kids.

They also move from crying, to a different-sounding crying to sometimes da-da-da-da-da.

And they know you, and they love you, and they get to know other people and sometimes they love them too, and you go 'NOOOO, ONLY LOVE ME!' but you can't keep them from the world and they start to need you a little less.

And that's great, because they're meant to become independent, but at the same time I feel, 'You needed me so much, I have never felt that needed before, and although it was horribly stressful for much of the time, in retrospect I'm forgetting the horribly stressful part and feeling sad that over time you will need me less and less.'

To my children, I am a constant.

And they will view me as I viewed my parents.

My parents, these people who never change, are, in my mind, the same as when I was small. The only time the illusion is broken is when they get ill, but then it's restored again once the crisis passes. They haven't changed, they're my parents, they are the same.

My children will view me in this way.

I may cut my hair or change its colour, swap my glasses, alter the way I dress, my weight, my make-up . . . Any of these things but I will be the same.

All of this while they will transform over and over in front of me. I will be introduced to a person I will have to get to know and they will greet me like an old friend (or enemy, depending) and I will wonder what it is they like now, who they like, where they've been, where they want to be, if they are happy.

Hoping they are.

Maybe then I can get out their old lemon dress, remember how small they used to be, have a bit of a cry and then f**k off to the bingo.

25 June

Last night was my first night away from the babies.

Ever.

I went to a wedding and I danced, and then I went to bed early because I can't function as a normal adult any more. I can't sleep in any more either – I woke up at 7.30 a.m.

And I missed the babies. Not because they're amazing in the morning, but because I was looking forward to seeing them.

I thought about how they both give this really happy squeal when I come to pick them up from crèche.

I thought, 'It's going to be like that, but it's going to be BIGGER! They're going to be really, really happy to see me.'

I turned the key in the door, opened it to find them both in the hall, and I said, 'Hi, babies!'

They turned, saw me and burst into tears.

They cried and they held up their arms because they wanted me to pick them up.

Both of them.

At the same time.

Two babies crying.

I was home.

27 June

Newborn babies have needs, which they like to express through the medium of having a good cry.

Their needs are fairly simple: 'Feed me, change me, wind me, change me again, maybe feed me again, I'm lonely, I'm tired, I've wind or maybe colic.'

Basically, wind/colic is usually the answer to 'I don't know why this child is still crying!'

As a new parent, my job was to fulfil those needs to the best of my ability, to make the crying stop, and to make the most of the intervening period of 'not crying' – or sleeping, as it's also known. They were simple times; simple and stressful times.

I obeyed the will of the baby and that was fine.

Now the babies are older, their needs still involve 'Feed me, change me, I'm tired' but 'wind/colic' has been replaced with teething. I'm fairly good at handling those needs but the babies have now thrown ridiculous 'wants' into the bargain, which they see as 'needs'.

'I need to pull my sister's hair.'

'I need to hold your phone and figure out what's going on with it.'

'I need to slap the cat.'

'I need to stay on this swing for about twenty days.'

'I need you to pick me up right now.'

'I need to be allowed to crawl on this floor covered in nails.'

Firstly, those aren't needs, you ridiculous kids. They're wants.

They can't understand why I won't fulfil them or why I actively stop them doing things.

'BUT YOU DID ALL THE OTHER THINGS I NEEDED.'

The babies are like musicians and I'm their manager. Back when they were starting out, they'd go to their gigs and need something simple – a chair, a plectrum, a glass of water. They'd do their thing, they'd get more famous and suddenly, their rider might include items such as 'a throne of gold, 20,000 plectra, water from a glacier'.

As their manager it's my job not to allow them to become so ridiculous that they lose sight of the music or venues no longer want to book them.

This involves saying 'no'.

At the moment, my big 'no' thing is them grabbing my glasses. I need my glasses to see, something which I have explained but now I say 'no'.

When I first say it, the babies smile. They think it's a game.

They try again.

'No.' This time in a firmer voice.

They laugh again, this is ridiculous, why would they not be allowed something they clearly want?

They try again.

'No.' Most firm voice, my brow is furrowed.

They look confused, then their brows furrow too. I am not obeying them. I should obey them. But I'm not.

Then they cry.

I get it, I really do. For months, all I have done is whatever they want; now they have to learn that sometimes what they want is f**king crazy.

This is a battle of wills, where I have to convince two babies that in fact, after months of them running the show, I run the show.

I'm taller, faster and stronger than them. They are smaller, slower and weaker but, oh god, so much louder than me.

I'm sure I could be louder if I tried, but I don't think them crying in the playground because they want to stay on the swing is best dealt with by me bellowing at the top of my lungs, 'GET THE F**K OFF THE SWING, YOU ARE BEING RIDICULOUS!'

Instead, I find myself talking to them as if I'm trying to defuse a hostage situation.

'I know you want to stay on the swing, but we have

to go home. You can come back tomorrow and the swing will still be here, if it isn't burnt down overnight.'

And it is hard.

Babies think that everything exists for them, and it's my job to crush that idea; for them to go from 'All of this is mine' to 'Adults get to do what they want, being a child sucks.'

So for the next few years, I guess this is it, a battle of wills, trying to teach them that 'You can't always get what you want, but if you cry sometimes, you might find you get what you need . . . Or we're asked to leave.'

2 July

The cat: the famous local celebrity.

The babies love her. They crawl towards her, then after her as she runs away. If she suddenly appears beside them, they stop crying.

'Cat' is one of the only words I'm confident they understand.

'Where is the cat?' And all eyes are on her.

We say 'cat', they say 'ka' or 'dat', or a number of different half-words as they try to get it right.

I don't even think they know I'm 'Mammy'.

The cat, for her part, likes to eat food they drop. She has nuzzled them individually on occasion, but gets alarmed if they crowd her – two babies crawling like zombies, arms outstretched to touch her. Although when the cat is actually within reach they get a little starstruck. First, they touch her ear delicately with one finger, or her whiskers. Bronagh babbles softly to her as she does this. Having actually touched her, they then get overzealous and try to either pull out a fistful of fur or pet her really hard.

I assume they intend to sell the fur to other fans of the cat on eBay.

So, basically they'd be selling it to each other. It

must be working for them because I'm constantly finding it on their clothes or in their mouths.

Don't eat your idols!

3 July

Colm wants to put an offer on the blue house which I still haven't seen. Meanwhile, we've been trying to make our house – which is currently rammed with baby things – a standard that it can be shown to people who want to buy it.

I arrange a viewing for the blue house and go on my own after work. I take a bus there and meet the estate agent outside. The house still has things in it belonging to the owner – she and her daughter still live there. The small things say this house belongs to a family but they have grown up. I think I like the house, but I am also convinced that it could be haunted. I no longer picture us in the houses we view because that's hoping for something that might not happen. But when I go back home I tell Colm to put in an offer.

4 July

Our offer on the blue house has been accepted.

'We could have a house?' I ask incredulously.

'If by "we" you mean "us and the bank", then yeah,' Colm replies.

He says we need to get a solicitor. Yet another person to add to the big mess of people involved in buying a house. I am happy, I think, but I've been so disappointed by the whole house-hunting thing that I won't believe we have a home until we have the keys in our hands. And I've checked that those keys actually open the door and aren't just fakes.

5 July

Ever meet someone who has the same model of phone you used to have?

'Oh, wow! Look at this! I used to have one just like it. That's a blast from the past. The one I have now is more advanced but I do kind of miss when they were simpler, and there was less messing around with them. Would you mind if I held it for a second? I won't do anything weird.'

Well, that's pretty much me with people who have babies younger than mine now.

9 July

It is a Saturday morning and we are getting ready to go on holiday.

6.20 a.m. Bronagh is awake. I know this because she's talking shite in her cot.

6.30 a.m. I bring her into our bed. She's putting her hand into my mouth to grab my tongue.

6.45 a.m. I tell Colm I'm going for a shower.

6.55 a.m. I'm back. Bronagh is complaining as Colm changes her nappy. Róisín is awake and pretty happy.

7.00 a.m. Colm decides he wants a shower. I stand Róisín in her cot so she's holding the side of it. Bronagh does the same in her own cot. They both do a thrusting dance, much like Mr Bean, while babbling.

7.10 a.m. I change Róisín's nappy.

7.15 a.m. The babies crawl on the floor while Colm and I get dressed. We pick out some spare clothes. He stays with the girls while I attempt to dry my hair. When I come back the babies are crying a lot. They are teething. The magic Calpol wand makes an appearance.

7.20 a.m. I try to sort out clothes for the babies to wear. I am taking vests out of their drawer and Bronagh is helping. She pulls out all of the vests. Then she pulls out all of the trousers. She isn't really helping.

7.30 a.m. Colm feeds the babies their Weetabix and I pack a bag with bottles and food and snacks. We make coffee and toast for us. The babies complain. They get a pancake each. Pieces are thrown on the floor a number of times. The cat eats it all. The babies reach for the cat like a crowd at a Beatles autograph signing.

7.50 a.m. I am attempting to wipe crusted Weetabix off their faces and hands. I ask Colm not to let it dry the next time. Both babies try to eat the facecloth.

8.00 a.m. Colm is dressing them.
'Oh, shit,' I say as a smell lets me know that I have left the hair straighteners on. I'm packing yet another bag with toys and bibs and such. I brush my teeth and hair while musing that maybe looking like hell when you're a mum means you're doing a good job.

8.15 a.m. The babies are back downstairs and I am still packing things. I suggest Colm brings the car closer to the house to load everything into it. As we are talking, we hear a thud behind us and crying.

8.20 a.m. I am holding Bronagh, who has stopped crying after falling over. A bump is beginning to appear on her forehead. I go to the shed to get ice out of the freezer. The ice looks very sorry for itself. It's now just a big lump of sadness where the potential for cocktails used to be.

I make a mental note to buy more ice – not for cocktails but because I expect more bumps.

8.24 a.m. I come back into the room to put the tea towel full of ice against Bronagh's forehead. Róisín is eating toilet roll. In fact, she isn't just eating it, she's relishing it. Now they're crawling, my most common question to them is 'What are you eating?' The answer is rarely something edible.

8.28 a.m. Colm is back from moving the car. Róisín pulls the fire guard away from the fireplace.
    'We need to leave!' I say, as chaos unfolds around me.

8.30 a.m. The babies are loaded into the buggy, crying the whining wail of the tired. Collectively, Colm and I carry six different-sized bags to the car.

8.40 a.m. The babies are loaded and we are ready to go to Donegal for a single night.
    A single night!
    Bloody hell.
    This parenting stuff is some craic.

15 July

Tomorrow the babies are one. Colm and I have been doing this parenting thing for almost a year. We each have a glass of wine, as if this is some end-of-year review for our company specializing in raising children. We congratulate each other on getting this far. It feels like an achievement and I have a small cry as a year's worth of emotions brush past me all at once.

16 July

It turns out that kids' birthdays are a lot of work for the parents. For the twins' first birthday, Colm did the BBQ and I did the baby wrangling and general 'does everyone have enough food?' enquiries while giving people too much food. This is a sure sign that I've gone full mammy.

My parents came and so did Colm's, and it was brilliant to be together for something when I didn't have postnatal depression.

I took photos but not as many as I'd have liked. A picture of the girls in their high chairs, wearing paper crowns the crèche had made them, under a banner I'd made announcing their names and age. It looked like the worst proof-of-age ID ever. Another photo of Colm's mum helping Bronagh to stand and my dad helping Róisín. The girls were wearing dresses slightly too big for them. They're size 12–18 months – they'll grow into them.

After the babies, the person I take the most photographs of is my mother, smiling, holding each baby in turn, rocking and singing to them, and happy. And a photo of us both, Bronagh between us, three generations brought together by cake and occasion and love. She tells me, 'You have two very happy babies.'

Being a parent has brought me closer to my mum, who has told me that 'I think it was better you had two babies at the same time. It gave you less time to worry about what you were doing wrong.' However, she also told me that we are doing an amazing job and that I am a natural mother. I don't know if such a thing exists, I'm just trying to find my own way and to make the best guesses. I'm realizing that my parents did the same, and that even though they weren't always right they managed to get me here.

And right now I am very happy.

17 July

Bronagh is in the baby bath for her weekly bath. There are bubbles all around her and it looks a bit like the old Cadbury's Flake advert. Except Bronagh isn't eating a chocolate bar, she's eating an orange rubber duck. She sees me looking at her and she grins into the duck, suds coating her fingers.

In the next room, Róisín is with Colm, waiting to get into the bath. She can't be in here with Bronagh because no chocolate advert ever involving a bath had another woman in the background, crying because she wanted her turn.

As Bronagh grins at me, I suddenly notice how she will be too big for the baby bath soon.

I remember newborn Bronagh crying beside a basin of water. I'm bearing the weight of her naked body as I run the wet cotton wool nervously over her face. She continues to cry. I am afraid I will drop her – her arms are spread wide, fingers too; they jerk uncontrollably because she cannot control them. I support her body in the basin of water, she continues to cry.

She stops crying when she is out of the basin.

Twelve months later, she is chewing a rubber duck and I am washing her with a facecloth while she sits there, happily kicking a large spray of suds and water at me. She supports herself in the bath of water, she continues to be happy.

She starts crying when she is out of the bath.

In the bedroom, she is wrapped in a towel and drinking milk from a bottle as I attempt to style her hair. I give her a mohawk, then curl the hair in my fingers. She drinks and watches me.

She is getting bigger and older.

'Remember this,' I tell myself. 'This right here – her lying on a changing table, wet hair, drinking milk, smiling at you periodically. This will go, things will change, she will get bigger, remember this.'

And I am staring intently, trying to absorb everything about this moment and to store it somewhere. Trying to enjoy her, in this quiet moment of her drinking milk, while being acutely aware that these things are transient.

'You will forget, you will forget. It doesn't matter, you will forget.'

Sadness wells and feels ridiculous because, as in a lucid dream, recognizing that this moment will end won't stop it from ending.

'You will forget.'

I take a photograph.

I don't want to.

But otherwise I will.

The photograph will go with the others. There are so many – all attempts to hold on to the time – to enjoy the babies in retrospect, how they changed.

Because now I realize the phrase 'Enjoy them, because it goes so fast' hurts.

Enjoying something because it is ending isn't enjoyable, because you get caught between the pressure to enjoy it and the knowledge that it will end.

And then the grief that it will be gone.

Which ruins the enjoyment.

You can't win.

This is the reason children keep their parents so busy. I'd rather be running around after them than worrying about the day that I will no longer have babies to run around after.

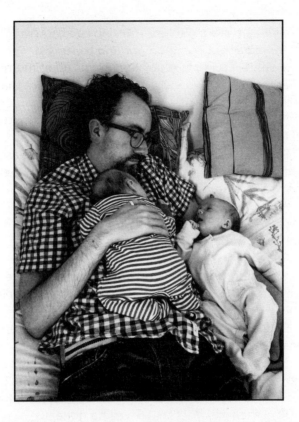

I wrote this about Colm on Father's Day. He wasn't meant to see it but I did show it to him. It's difficult for me to express how much he means to me, but hopefully by now you understand something of how much he does. And why the last part of this book should be about him.

I am asking him how he is.
    'Tired. How are you?'
    'Pregnant,' I say.
    He is delighted.
    I am lying on a hospital bed.
    Shivering uncontrollably, my teeth are chattering.
    We are here because they said we needed to come in.

Because a test I took because of a bleed said I needed to be scanned.

My teeth chatter, I cannot speak; I am scared, nervous and excited.

He is concerned. He holds my hand.

I am scanned.

It is twins.

He is shocked.

He is delighted.

I am sitting on the floor beside the toilet.

There is a towel there so I am comfortable.

I tell him I don't understand why people go through this.

I tell him we have to leave; the smell of the bacon he cooked is too bad. He hands me a glass of water.

We leave.

He does not cook anything that smells for weeks.

I look in the mirror.

I announce that I just look fat.

I pat my stomach.

'I look fat.'

'Not fat. Pregnant, Maria,' he says.

'The babies are moving, put your hand here.'

He does; he feels them move.

He begins nightly 'baby inspections'.

Putting his hand on my tummy, he says, 'Hmm-hmm, hmm-hmm, yes, there are babies in there.'

He does this to a bigger and bigger belly.

He puts his head against my stomach.

He says he can hear a heartbeat.

He does this every time I get worried that they aren't kicking.

They are kicking too hard, I complain then too.

In the dark, I am crying.

'I am afraid to be a parent, I can barely look after myself.'

'It will be fine, we can do this,' he says.

I am less afraid.

I am in labour.

'What do I do?' I ask.

'Push against your bum,' they say.

I push everything. I am tired, I am thirsty.

He squirts water into my mouth between contractions.

I turn to him with my mouth open, he sprays water in it.

I ask him not to look at the baby coming out.

He does – the first baby comes out.

He holds her; he is holding her against his skin and I am pushing again.

I am home from hospital.

He is experiencing his first sleepless night.

Feeds every three hours.

I am feeding a baby.

He is feeding a baby.

We are taking turns in the 'good chair' and the 'shit chair' to do it.

I am holding a crying baby.

He is holding a crying baby.

We are trying to watch *The Good Wife* in the bedroom at 9 p.m.

We are eating toast at 5 a.m.

I am waking every time they stir in their sleep.

He is not.

'They're awake,' I say.

We both get up.

He is changing a nappy.

He is changing a nappy.

He is changing a nappy.

He is changing a nappy, the poo is everywhere.

He is humming the theme from *Platoon*.

He is getting puked on.

He is getting puked on.

He is getting puked on.

He is asking why they always seem to puke on him.

I am singing '(I Just) Died in Your Arms Tonight' and manipulating the baby's mouth to sing at Colm and the other baby.

'She is loving that,' he says.

She is smiling for the first time.

He gets to see it.

I am in a room and both babies are crying.

I am on my own.

He comes home and I burst into tears.

He takes over, I leave.

He is telling me he lost his job.

He is looking for work.

He is looking for work.

He is holding a baby and looking for work.

I am crying in the park.

'I don't know why I am crying.'

He is encouraging me to see my GP.

'I don't want to have postnatal depression.'

He is concerned.

He hugs me.

I cannot feel it.

I am telling him I want to go back to work.

He is arranging to go part time in his new job so one of us is home with the kids.

I cannot go part time.

He spends Mondays and Fridays with the babies on his own.

We are getting ready for work.

We are dressing a baby each.

They are crying.

'I have to leave to go to work,' I say.

I kiss him goodbye, I kiss them goodbye.

He takes them to crèche.

He is blowing on a baby's belly.

He is waving a baby's legs as it giggles.

He is having a baby pull at his beard.

264

He is saying, 'Look, babies, it's the famous local celebrity: the cat.'

He is carrying a baby and the changing bag into the toilet.

He is singing 'Row, Row, Row Your Boat.'

He is making Ready Brek and asking if we have any fruit to put in it for the babies.

He is accompanying them as they crawl into the kitchen.

He is lifting the cat's bowl out of the way.

He is putting them in high chairs.

He is trying to feed the babies.

He is wiping food out of a baby's ear.

He is washing a baby.

He is washing bottles.

He is scooping milk into bottles.

He is pouring milk into a baby.

He is saying 'da-da da-da da-da'.

They are saying 'da-da-da-da-da-da-da-da'.

He is unwrapping a gift.

'It's from the babies.'

It is socks.

I am saying 'Happy Father's Day.'

I am
    Not saying enough.

ACKNOWLEDGEMENTS

Firstly, I need to admit that when I was writing all of these small diary entries I never thought that they would somehow end up in a book. If I had, I probably wouldn't have sworn as much as I do.

I would like to thank my agent, Faith O'Grady, for asking 'What sort of book do you want to write?', and for talking sense when it was needed. Thanks to everyone at Transworld (Ireland and UK) for guiding me through this, especially Fiona Murphy for allowing this book to evolve from 'a book of cartoons' to something more personal, and Michelle Signore for editing it into something that resembles a book and allaying my panic and laughing at my jokes. I'd also like to thank Rebecca Wright for her copy-editing and for our entire interaction being on the comments section in the margins of a document.

A huge thank you is due to my friends with whom my panicked thoughts and reflections on parenting were shared. Thank you for your good humour in my repeated uploading of pictures of my children, and for telling me that it would be OK – and for also not saying that when it wasn't needed. I'd love to give big thanks to Shaun for all of his love and support and for showing me that kids don't have to be blood to be family.

Thanks to all of the parents in the IMBA for being a sounding board, a place of good fun and for allowing me to see children I do not know grow up alongside my own. And to the twin mothers Jackie and Sarah for deciding that having twins is crazy but for also keeping me sane and having a sense of humour. Thanks to Emma, Anna and Brenda for journeying to parenthood with me and letting me vent on a Monday morning.

I'm grateful to the people I've been lucky enough to

work with, especially those who encouraged me to do this. I want to give a special mention to my work-wife, Aoife, for being a sounding board for pieces I'd written, for her excellent humour and for helping me brainstorm names for this book – 'What about *Jaws*?' . . .

A big thank you, too, to all of the people in my life who ended up in this book because of our interactions, associations and acquaintance. Thanks to my counsellor and my GP for looking after me without judgement and always with compassion and kindness. And to all of the child-care workers who looked after my kids and continue to do so with love, laughter and good humour – thank you for being part of our lives.

And a huge amount of thanks and much love to our families: my parents for showing me who parents are and how they can be, for their help, common sense and dark humour, and Colm's family for more of the same.

I couldn't have done this without Colm, literally and emotionally. Hopefully he knows how much he means to me and forgives me for the panicked frustrations around trying to get everything done. Thank you for coming on this amazing adventure with me.

Finally, to my babies – you will always be my babies even when it feels really inappropriate for me to say that. Thanks for coming along and letting us be your guides to the start of this big journey that is life and for finally sleeping though the night.

MARIA BOYLE was born in Donegal and ended up in Dublin to complete a PhD in science. She now lives in Dublin with her husband, one-eyed cat and identical twin girls. Although a (possibly) respected scientist, she is better known as the cartoonist Twisteddoodles. Twisteddoodles started by accident in the hope of marrying her love of jokes with her ability to draw a discernible face. Her work has appeared all over the world and has been translated into many different languages. Twisteddoodles' cartoons are inspired by her real-life adventures and cover areas such as science, coffee, news events, modern life and, more recently, parenting. You can find her on Facebook, Twitter and Instagram as @Twisteddoodles and sometimes you can find her in a supermarket asking her children not to touch everything.